ONCOLOGY NURSING

*An Essential Guide
for Patient Care*

ONCOLOGY NURSING

An Essential Guide for Patient Care

Christine Miaskowski, RN, PhD, FAAN

Associate Professor and Chair
Department of Physiological Nursing
University of California
San Francisco, California

W.B. SAUNDERS COMPANY
A Division of Harcourt Brace & Company
Philadelphia • London • Toronto • Montreal • Sydney • Tokyo

W.B. SAUNDERS COMPANY
A Division of Harcourt Brace & Company

The Curtis Center
Independence Square West
Philadelphia, Pennsylvania 19106

Library of Congress Cataloging-in-Publication Data

Miaskowski, Christine.
    Oncology nursing: an essential guide for patient care / Christine
Miaskowski.

        p.   cm.

    ISBN 0–7216–6041–X

    1. Cancer—Nursing.   I. Title.
    [DNLM: 1. Oncologic Nursing—methods.   2. Neoplasms—nursing.
3. Antineoplastic Agents.   4. HIV Infections—complications.   WY
156 M6180 1997]

    RC266.M53 1997   610.73′698—dc20

DNLM/DLC   96-19932

ONCOLOGY NURSING: AN ESSENTIAL GUIDE FOR PATIENT CARE   ISBN 0–7216–6041–X

Printed in the United States of America.

Last digit is the print number: 9   8   7   6   5   4   3   2   1

This book is dedicated to my nephew and godson,
John Patrick Connolly.
This precious child inspires me to live a life of joy and peace.

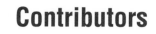

Contributors

Several of my students who graduated from the Oncology Nursing Master's Program at the University of California, San Francisco in 1995 contributed sections to this book.

Kathryn M. Barrett, RN, MS
CNS, Pediatric Oncology,
University of California, San Francisco,
San Francisco, California
- Osteogenic sarcoma
- Wilms' tumor

Rose Campbell, RN, MS
Research Clinician,
AIDS Research Consortium
of Atlanta, Atlanta,
Georgia
- Non–small-cell lung cancer
- Small-cell lung cancer

Donna Griesbach, RN, MS
Research Coordinator,
University of Louisville,
Louisville, Kentucky
- Ovarian cancer: epithelial
- Pancreatic cancer

Christopher Hawkins, RN, MS
Research Nurse, University of California,
San Francisco, San Francisco, California
- Testicular cancer: nonseminoma
- Testicular cancer: seminomas

Luisa P. Kelly, RN, MS
Nurse in Private Practice,
Santa Cruz, California
- Bladder cancer: invasive
- Bladder cancer: superficial

Lisa A. Kragness, RN, MS
Rancho Cucamonga,
California
- Kidney cancer: renal cell carcinoma
- Prostate cancer

Kazuko Onishi, RN, MS
Professor, College of
Medical Sciences, Mie
University, Mie, Japan
- Gallbladder cancer
- Stomach cancer

Kathy Roegner, RN, MS
Nurse Practitioner,
Primary Practice,
Veterans Administration Outpatient Clinic,
Oakland, California
- Malignant melanoma
- Thyroid cancer

Enny R. Zimmer, RN, MS
Home Care Nurse,
Valley Care Home Health,
Livermore, California
- Chronic lymphocytic leukemia
- Multiple myeloma

Preface

This book makes a unique contribution to the oncology and HIV nursing literature. The format and design of the book enable it to be used as a quick reference guide by nurses caring for patients with cancer or HIV disease in inpatient and outpatient settings. Each page of the book gives an at-a-glance review of a specific clinical condition, patient problem, or pharmacologic agent.

The book is organized into seven sections, A to G. The first four sections provide information on various aspects of the management of patients with cancer. The last three sections focus on the care of patients with HIV disease.

Section A provides at-a-glance information on over 60 different oncologic diagnoses. On a single page, nurses can review the epidemiology of the cancer as well as specific etiologies and risk factors associated with the disease. For a given cancer, the most common signs and symptoms of the disease, the major diagnostic tests employed, the most common metastatic sites, and the most common treatment strategies are outlined. In addition, the most common patient problems, potential oncologic emergencies, and prognosis for each disease are reviewed.

The list of cancer diagnoses is very specific. For example, two types of bladder cancer (i.e., superficial and invasive) are included in the text. This level of detail gives nurses the necessary information to provide the most comprehensive and specific care possible.

Section B provides one-page references for over fifty of the most common problems associated with cancer or cancer treatment. Each of the one-page references provides a definition of the problem, a list of etiologies or risk factors, the most common assessment parameters, and the test used most often to diagnose the problem. In addition, the most commonly used pharmacologic and nonpharmacologic approaches to managing the problem are outlined. A list of the most-encountered common potential problems associated with a given problem is also provided. Nurses can use this section independently to manage specific patient problems or cross-reference this section with the section on specific cancers to develop a nursing management plan for problems given patients may develop as a result of their disease or treatment.

Section C of the book provides a readily available source of information on the most common chemotherapeutic agents and biologics that are administered to oncology patients. Information provided on each pharmacologic agent includes the agent's classification and mechanism of action; the most common cancers treated by the agent; the most common dosing schedules and routes of administration; the side-effects associated with the agent; and special considerations nurses need to know when administering these agents. Again, this section can easily be cross-referenced with Sections A and B.

Section D, related to the management of oncology patients, provides at-a-glance reference for eighteen of the most common oncologic emergencies. Each single-page reference provides information on the prevalence of the emergency, the most common etiologies and risk factors, the most common signs and symptoms associated with emergency, and the most commonly ordered diagnostic tests. The treatment of the condition is outlined as are the potential problems associated with the oncologic emergency that require nursing care.

The last three sections of the book are designed to facilitate the nursing management of patients with HIV disease. The most common AIDS-related conditions are summarized. In addition, the most common problems associated with HIV disease or treatment and the most common pharmacologic agents administered to this population of patients are described. Again, nurses caring for patients with HIV disease will find these sections extremely useful in developing a comprehensive nursing management plan.

Another outstanding feature of this book is the comprehensive bibliography at the end of each section. The most current review articles on a given topic are listed in the bibliography. Nurses who need more detailed information on a particular topic will find these review articles extremely useful.

Oncology Nursing: An Essential Guide for Patient Care should be used as a quick reference guide *while caring* for oncology patients or patients with HIV disease. Nurses can consult the text while caring for or teaching patients about their disease and treatment. By using this one-page reference, nurses can be sure that they are performing comprehensive assessments of their patients and including all of the necessary components in their teaching and management plans.

Christine Miaskowski, RN, PhD, FAAN

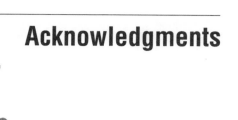

Acknowledgments

Nothing that we do is done in isolation, and this book is no exception. Numerous people contributed their time and talents to making this project a success. I would like to thank the graduate students in the Oncology Master's Program at the University of California, San Francisco, who provided contributions to this book. In addition, I would like to express my appreciation to Barbara Nelson Cullen, my nursing editor at the W. B. Saunders Company, who provided me with numerous hours of inspiration, guidance, and "pearls of wisdom." Barbara's friendship and support made the development and completion of this book a truly enjoyable experience. Finally, I need to express my sincerest thanks and appreciation to Julie Alden. Julie is an exceptionally talented individual who spent countless hours typing and formatting this book. I am deeply grateful for her expertise, support, and attention to detail. Without Julie, this book would never have been a reality.

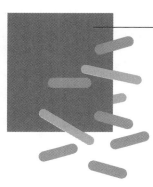

Contents

Specific Cancers

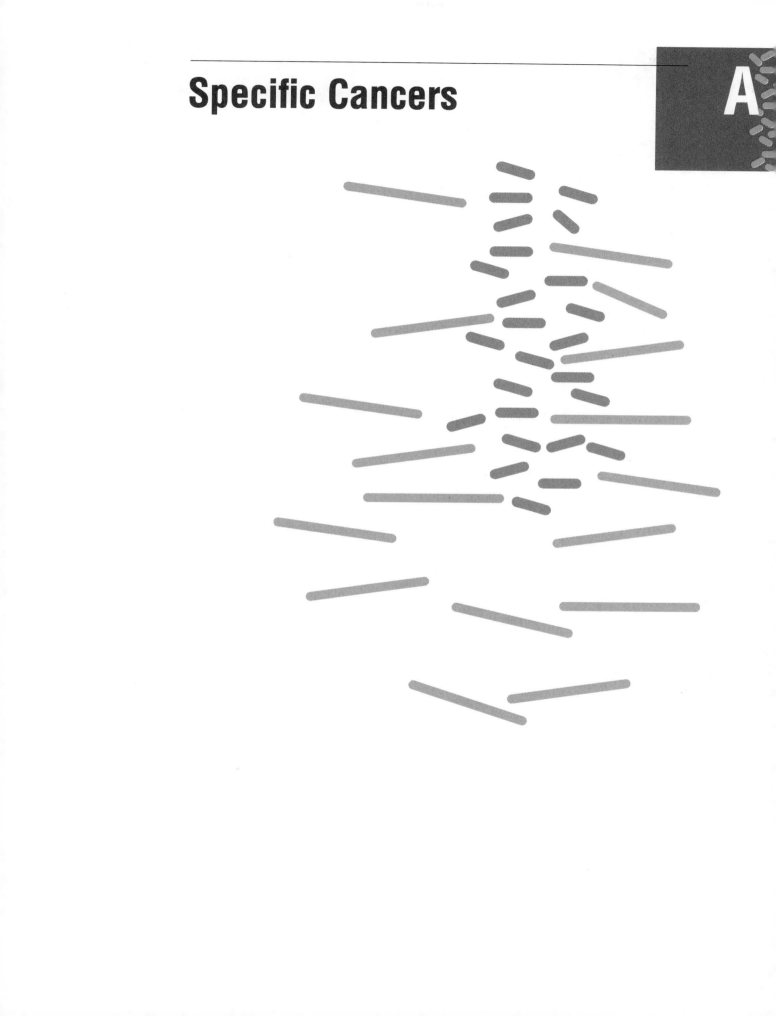

Anal Cancer

Epidemiology
- 1–2% of all anorectal cancers
- Incidence increasing in male homosexual population
- Male-female ratio 2.2:1

Etiology/Risk Factors
- Chronic perianal disease
- Presence of genital condylomas
- Receptive anal intercourse
- Human papillomavirus
- Cervical cancer
- Cigarette smoking
- Organ transplant patients

Signs and Symptoms
- Bleeding
- Discharge
- Itching
- Pain following defecation
- Rectal mass
- Tenderness on palpation

Diagnostic Tests
- Abdominal ultrasound
- Anoscopy
- CT of abdomen and pelvis
- Chest radiography
- CBC
- Digital rectal examination
- Liver function tests
- Serum creatinine

Metastatic Sites
- Bone
- Brain
- Liver
- Lung
- Lymph nodes
- Retroperitoneum

Treatment

- Surgery: small tumors can be surgically excised; abdominoperineal resection indicated if chemotherapy and radiation therapy are not successful
- Radiation therapy and chemotherapy (5-FU/mitomycin and pelvic radiation) successful in 80–90% of patients with local disease

Potential Problems
- Abdominal ascites
- Anxiety
- Cystitis
- Diarrhea
- Fecal incontinence
- Fistulas
- Impaired sexual functioning
- Mood disturbances
- Nutritional deficit
- Pain
- Perianal skin lesions
- Pruritus

Potential Oncologic Emergencies
- Intestinal obstruction
- Pathologic fractures
- Septic shock
- Spinal cord compression

Prognosis
- 5-year relapse-free survival with combination therapy 62–86%

Astrocytoma

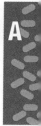

Epidemiology

- Accounts for 30–40% of childhood CNS tumors
- Half of tumors in cerebral hemispheres; other half in the thalamus, hypothalamus, third ventricle, and basal ganglia
- Male-female ratio 2:1

Etiology/Risk Factors

- Children with leukemia treated with radiation therapy as prophylaxis for CNS disease
- Genetic defect

Signs and Symptoms

- General manifestations
  - Headache
  - Mental status changes
  - Papilledema
  - Pupillary changes
  - Seizures
  - Vasomotor and autonomic changes
  - Vomiting
- Focal manifestations (depend on the location of the tumor)
- Changes in cognitive functioning
- Gait disturbance
- Hearing impairments
- Meningeal signs
- Motor impairment
- Neuroendocrine disturbances
- Paresthesias
- Personality changes
- Visual changes

Diagnostic Tests

- Biopsy
- CT
- PET
- MRI

Metastatic Sites

- None

Treatment

- Surgical resection is the primary therapy
- Radiation therapy may be useful in patients > 40 years of age with more extensive tumors

Potential Problems

- Bradycardia
- Decreased mobility
- Impaired cognition
- Ineffective breathing pattern
- Mood disturbance
- Nausea and vomiting
- Pain
- Potential for injury
- Self-care deficit
- Sensory-perceptual deficit

Potential Oncologic Emergencies

- Increased intracranial pressure
- Respiratory arrest

Prognosis

- Low-grade tumors are associated with long-term survival rate of 80%
- Grade III tumors are associated with 50%, 3-year survival rate, and Grade IV tumors with 15–20%, 3-year survival

Bladder Cancer: Invasive

Epidemiology
- 16,800 new cases per year
- 1% of all cancers
- Male-female ratio 4:1

Etiology/Risk Factors
- Age >50
- Cigarette smoking
- Exposure to cyclophosphamide
- History of abusing phenacetin
- History of superficial bladder tumors
- History of urinary conditions
- Living in urban areas
- Occupational exposure to dye, rubber, or leather
- Previous pelvic irradiation

Signs and Symptoms
- Early: hematuria, frequency, urgency, painful or difficult urination
- Late: flank, rectal, or pelvic pain; changes in bowel habits; lower extremity edema; weight loss; anorexia; fever

Diagnostic Tests
- Bimanual examination
- Bladder washings for cytology and flow cytometry
- Bone scan
- Chest radiography
- CBC
- Chemistry profile
- CT of abdomen and pelvis
- Cystoscopy with transurethral biopsy
- IVP/excretory urography
- MRI of abdomen, rectum, and pelvis
- Urinalysis

Metastatic Sites
- Bone
- Liver
- Lung
- Regional lymph nodes

Treatment

- Surgery: radical cystectomy with or without pelvic node dissection as curative therapy
- Radiation therapy, alone or with chemotherapy, in patients who are not surgical candidates
- Chemotherapy, used for metastatic disease, adjuvant and neoadjuvant therapy
  - Cisplatin (70 mg/m^2 IV) every 3 weeks
  - Methotrexate (40 mg/m^2 IV) weekly ± leucovorin
  - Doxorubicin (45–75 mg/m^2 IV) every 3 weeks
  - Vinblastine (0.10–0.15 mg/m^2 IV) weekly
- Combination therapy:
  - CMV: cisplatin (100 mg/m^2 IV on day 1) + methotrexate (30 mg/m^2, IV on days 1, 8) + vinblastine (4 mg/m^2 IV on days 1, 8) every 21 days
  - MVAC: methotrexate (30 mg/m^2 IV on days 1, 15, 22) + vinblastine (3 mg/m^2 IV on day 2, 15, 22) + doxorubicin (30 mg/m^2 IV on day 2) + cisplatin (70 mg/m^2 IV on day 2) every 21 days
  - CISCA: cisplatin (100 mg/m^2 IV on day 2) + doxorubicin (50 mg/m^2 IV on day 1) + cyclophosphamide (650 mg/m^2 IV on day 1) every 21 days

Potential Problems
- Alteration in urinary elimination
- Changes in body image
- Chemotherapy-induced toxicities
- Infection
- Pain
- Periostomal skin breakdown
- Radical cystectomy
- Sexual dysfunction

Potential Oncologic Emergencies
- Cardiopulmonary arrest
- Septic shock
- Uremia

Prognosis
- Using AJCC/UICC system, 5-year survival: Stage II, 55%; Stage III, 20–35%; Stage IV, <5%

Bladder Cancer: Superficial

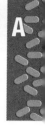

Epidemiology
- 33,600 new cases per year
- 3% of all cancers
- Male-female ratio 4:1

Etiology/Risk Factors
- Cigarette smoking
- Exposure to cyclophosphamide
- History of phenacetin abuse
- History of urinary tract conditions
- Living in urban areas
- Occupational exposure to dye, rubber, or leather
- Previous pelvic irradiation

Signs and Symptoms
- Early: hematuria, urgency, frequency, painful micturition, difficulty passing urine, recurrent infections of the urinary tract
- Late: flank, rectal, or pelvic pain; changes in bowel habits; lower extremity edema; weight loss; anorexia; fever

Diagnostic Tests
- Bimanual examination
- Bladder washings for cytology and flow cytometry
- CBC
- Chemistry profile
- Cystoscopy with transurethral biopsy
- IVP/excretory urography
- Urinalysis

Metastatic Sites
- None: tumor confined to the mucosa

Treatment

- Surgery: TURBT with fulguration as a curative resection; segmental cystectomy (rarely indicated); radical cystectomy (in selected patients with extensive superficial involvement)
- Radiation therapy primarily for patients who are not candidates for surgery
- Intravesical chemotherapy or immunotherapy: prophylactic measure after TUR or employed prior to forms of treatment other than TUR in patients with multiple tumors; intravesical therapy is accomplished by instilling drug into the bladder, repositioning the patient, and draining the drug out 1–2 hours later
  - BCG (1 ampule diluted in 50 ml saline) at weekly intervals beginning shortly after resection and lasting 6–10 weeks; treatment of choice for CIS
  - Thiotepa (30 or 60 mg) weekly for 4–6 weeks
  - Mitomycin C (20–40 mg) weekly for 8 weeks
  - Doxorubicin (50 mg) weekly for 6–8 weeks
  - Epirubicin (30–80 mg) weekly for 8 weeks
  - Ethoglucid (1 or 2% solution) weekly for 4–56 weeks

Potential Problems
- Altered urinary elimination
- Cystitis
- Infection
- Pain

Potential Oncologic Emergencies
- Septic shock

Prognosis
- Using AJCC/UICC system, 5-year survival: Stage 0, 90%; Stage I, 75%

Breast Cancer: Early Invasive Disease

Epidemiology
- 75% of patients with newly diagnosed breast cancer have tumors < 5 cm diameter

Etiology/Risk Factors
- Increasing age
- High-fat "Western" diet
- Family history
- Early menarche
- Late menopause
- History of breast cancer
- History of benign breast disease
- Mutations in specific genes (BRCA1 and BRCA2)

Signs and Symptoms
- Painless mass or lump in the breast
- Persistent dermatitis of nipple or areola
- Serous or bloody nipple discharge

Diagnostic Tests
- Bone scan
- Chest radiography
- CBC
- Hormone receptor assays for estrogen and progesterone
- Liver scan
- Mammography

Metastatic Sites
- Bone
- Brain
- Liver
- Lymph nodes

Treatment

- Surgery: modified radical mastectomy or node excision followed by radiation therapy
- Axillary dissection: (a valuable staging procedure for most patients)
- Adjuvant chemotherapy or hormonal therapy is recommended for patients with node-positive disease
  - For premenopausal women, the recommended therapy is CAF: cyclophosphamide (100 mg/m^2 PO daily on days 1–14); doxorubicin (30 mg/m^2 IV push on days 1 and 8); 5-FU (600 mg/m^2 IV on days 1 and 8); and prednisone (40 mg/m^2 PO on days 1 to 14) repeat every 28 days for 6 cycles
  - For postmenopausal women, the recommended therapy is tamoxifen (10 mg PO b.i.d. for at least 2 years)

Potential Problems
- Anxiety
- Body image disturbance
- Fear
- Impaired sexual functioning
- Infection
- Lymphedema
- Pain

Potential Oncologic Emergencies
- Abdominal ascites
- Brachial plexopathy
- Hypercalcemia
- Pathologic fractures
- Pericardial effusions
- Pleural effusions
- Radiation pneumonitis
- Septic shock
- Spinal cord compression

Prognosis
- Prognosis varies depending on age, tumor size, hormone receptor status, axillary node status, histologic subtype, and tumor grade

Breast Cancer: Locally Advanced Disease

Epidemiology

- Heterogeneous group of malignancies

Etiology/Risk Factors

- Increasing age
- High-fat "Western" diet
- Family history
- Early menarche
- Late menopause
- History of breast cancer
- History of benign breast disease
- Mutations in specific genes (BRCA1 and BRCA2)

Signs and Symptoms

- Painless mass or lump in the breast
- Tumor > 5 cm with mobile axillary nodes
- Tumor of any size with fixed axillary or clinically enlarged internal mammary nodes
- Tumor with direct extension to the chest wall and/or skin
- Inflammatory cancer, with or without nodal involvement

Diagnostic Tests

- Bone scan
- Chest radiography
- CBC
- Hormone receptor assays for estrogen and progesterone
- Liver scan
- Mammography

Metastatic Sites

- Bone
- Brain
- Liver
- Lymph nodes

Treatment

- Multimodal therapy is recommended for all patients; the sequence of treatment (i.e., chemotherapy, surgery, radiation therapy) is largely dependent on the operability of the primary tumor
- Bone marrow transplantation

Potential Problems

- Alteration in mobility
- Anxiety
- Body image disturbance
- Fear
- Impaired sexual functioning
- Infection
- Lymphedema
- Pain

Potential Oncologic Emergencies

- Abdominal ascites
- Brachial plexopathy
- GVHD
- Hypercalcemia
- Pathologic fractures
- Pericardial effusions
- Pleural effusions
- Radiation pneumonitis
- Septic shock
- Spinal cord compression

Prognosis

- Complete response rates at the time of surgery are 58–100%; 3- to 5-year relapse-free survival in 20–73%; local recurrence rates are 13–38%

Breast Cancer: Noninvasive Disease

Epidemiology

- Lobular CIS (LCIS)
  - Discovered in association with another indicator for biopsy
  - 90% of patients are premenopausal
  - 1–2% prevalence in the general population
  - Decreased incidence after menopause
- Ductal CIS (DCIS)
  - Peak incidence ages 51–59 years
  - Constitutes 5% of male breast cancer

Etiology/Risk Factors

- Increasing age
- High-fat "Western" diet
- Family history
- Early menarche
- Late menopause
- History of breast cancer
- History of benign breast disease
- Mutations in specific genes (BRCA1 and BRCA2)

Signs and Symptoms

- LCIS
  - Multifocal, multicentric, or bilateral
  - More often associated with infiltrating carcinoma of lobular or tubular histology
  - Impalpable; incidental finding at biopsy
- DCIS
  - Finding on mammography
  - Palpable mass

Diagnostic Tests

- Biopsy
- Mammography
- Hormone receptor assays for estrogen and progesterone

Metastatic Sites

- Bone
- Brain
- Liver
- Lymph nodes

Treatment

- LCIS: simple excision with observation; ipsilateral mastectomy without axillary dissection and with biopsy of the contralateral breast; or bilateral total mastectomy
- DCIS: excision with clear margins, making sure all microcalcifications are removed; excision followed by breast irradiation; or traditional total mastectomy with reconstruction

Potential Problems

- Anxiety
- Body image disturbance
- Fear
- Impaired sexual functioning
- Pain

Potential Oncologic Emergencies

- Abdominal ascites
- Hypercalcemia
- Pathologic fractures
- Pericardial effusions
- Pleural effusions
- Spinal cord compression

Prognosis

- LCIS: over 10-year follow-up, recurrence was 2.7% and mortality 0.9%
- DCIS: 5-year event-free survival was 84.4% in an irradiated group, as compared with 73.8% in an excision-alone group

Burkitt's Lymphoma

Epidemiology

- Endemic regions include equatorial Africa and New Guinea
- Peak age 5–8 years in the United States
- Incidence 0.1–0.3 per 100,000 children
- Male-female ratio 2.3:1.0

Etiology/Risk Factors

- Epstein-Barr virus
- Congenital immunodeficiency disorders

Signs and Symptoms

- Abdominal mass
- Ascites
- Intussusception
- Intestinal obstruction
- Intestinal perforation

Diagnostic Tests

- Abdominal ultrasound
- BUN
- Bone marrow biopsy
- Chest radiography
- History and physical examination
- Level of β_2-microglobulins
- Lumbar puncture
- Serum uric acid level
- Serum LDH level

Metastatic Sites

- Bone marrow
- CNS

Treatment

- Treatment depends on stage of disease
- Prevent tumor lysis syndrome with adequate hydration and urate oxydase
- Administer chemotherapy: one common regimen is COMP: vincristine (1 mg/m^2 IV on day 1); cyclophosphamide (300 mg/m^2 IV on day 1); prednisone (2 mg/kg IV on days 1 to 7); methotrexate (15 mg/m^2 IT on day 1) with 5 to 7 days' rest
- Bone marrow transplantation

Potential Problems

- Depression
- Fatigue
- Fluid volume deficit
- High risk for injury
- Infection
- Mucositis
- Nausea and vomiting
- Nutritional deficit
- Pain

Potential Oncologic Emergencies

- Septic shock
- Tumor lysis syndrome

Prognosis

- Treatment produces 90% complete response rate with 60–90% long-term survival in patients with Stage III or IV disease

CNS Lymphoma

Epidemiology
- Tumor presents as a solitary or multifocal parenchymal brain mass
- Most tumors are B-cell lymphomas

Etiology/Risk Factors
- AIDS
- Congenital immunodeficiencies
- Transplant recipient

Signs and Symptoms
- General manifestations
  - Headache
  - Mental status changes
  - Papilledema
  - Seizures
  - Vasomotor and autonomic changes
  - Vomiting
- Focal manifestations (depend on location of the tumor)
  - Changes in cognitive functioning
  - Gait disturbances
  - Hearing impairment
  - Meningeal signs
  - Motor impairments
  - Neuroendocrine disturbances
  - Paresthesias
  - Personality changes
  - Visual changes

Diagnostic Tests
- Biopsy
- CSF examination
- CT
- MRI

Metastatic Sites
- Leptomeninges
- Spinal cord

Treatment
- Common management is to deliver two or three cycles of chemotherapy (e.g., high-dose methotrexate, cytosine arabinoside) with intrathecal methotrexate, followed by whole-brain irradiation

Potential Problems
- Bradycardia
- Decreased mobility
- Impaired cognition
- Ineffective breathing pattern
- Mood disturbance
- Nausea and vomiting
- Pain
- Potential for injury
- Self-care deficit
- Sensory-perceptual deficit

Potential Oncologic Emergencies
- Increased intracranial pressure
- Respiratory arrest
- Spinal cord compression

Prognosis
- Overall median survival approximately 1 year

Cervical Cancer

Epidemiology
- Third most common cancer of the female genital tract
- Approximately 15,000 new cases per year
- Approximately 4600 deaths per year
- Approximately 80% of the tumors are squamous cell

Etiology/Risk Factors
- Early age at first coitus
- Early child bearing
- Multiple sex partners
- Prostitution
- Venereal infection
- Contact with high-risk males
- Cigarette smoking
- Pelvic irradiation
- Low socioeconomic status
- Immunodeficiency
- Vitamin A and C deficiencies
- Oral contraceptive use
- Human papillomavirus infection

Signs and Symptoms
- Irregular bleeding
- Low back pain
- Malodorous vaginal discharge
- Obstructive uropathy
- Palpable supraclavicular or groin nodes
- Postcoital bleeding
- Postmenopausal bleeding
- Vaginal bleeding
- Weight loss

Diagnostic Tests
- Barium enema
- CBC
- CT
- Chest radiography
- Colposcopy
- Cystoscopy
- Endocervical curettage
- Excisional or cone biopsy
- Intravenous pyelogram
- MRI
- Proctoscopy
- Serum chemistries

Metastatic Sites
- Bladder
- Lung
- Kidney and ureters
- Rectum
- Regional lymph nodes

Treatment
- Treatment determined by stage of disease
- Surgical approach depends on stage of disease: excisional conization or extrafascial hysterectomy; modified radical or radical hysterectomy; partial exenteration
- Radiation doses are tailored to the tumor volume (range 4000–6000 cGy)
- Chemotherapy traditionally reserved for patients with nonresectable or metastatic disease; active agents are cisplatin (50–75 mg/m^2 IV), carboplatin, ifosfamide, methotrexate, mitomycin, and vinblastine

Potential Problems
- Abdominal cramps
- Abdominal pain
- Altered body image
- Cystitis
- Diarrhea
- Dyspareunia
- Fibrosis of irradiated organs/tissues
- Fistulas
- Lymphedema
- Nausea and vomiting
- Proctitis
- Sexual dysfunction
- Urinary frequency
- Vaginal stenosis

Potential Oncologic Emergencies
- Intestinal obstruction
- Obstructive uropathy
- Pleural effusions
- Sepsis
- Spinal cord compression

Prognosis
- Cure rates: approximately 80% for Stage I disease, 60% for Stage II, 30% for Stage III, and 10% for Stage IV

Colon Cancer

Epidemiology
- 155,000 new cases per year
- 15% of all cancers
- Male-female ratio 1:1

Etiology/Risk Factors
- Age > 40 years
- Familial polyposis coli
- High-fat, low-fiber diet
- History of breast or genital cancer in females
- History of colorectal polyps
- Inflammatory bowel disease
- Family history

Signs and Symptoms
- Early: none or nonspecific ones
- Late: change in bowel habits, abdominal pain, melena, weight loss

Diagnostic Tests
- Air-contrast barium enema
- CBC
- Colonoscopy
- LFTs
- Serum CEA
- Stool guaiac

Metastatic Sites
- Bone
- Liver
- Lungs

Treatment
- Surgery: partial colectomy for curative resection
- Radiation therapy: primarily for persons at high risk for local recurrence
- Adjuvant chemotherapy
  - Leucovorin (20 mg/m^2 IV) + 5-FU (425 mg/m^2 IV) $\times$ 5 days
  - Methotrexate (200 mg/m^2 IV) + 5-FU (600 mg/m^2 IV) + leucovorin (10 mg/m^2 PO, q6hr for 6 doses), repeat every 2 weeks
  - 5-FU (750 mg/m^2 IV infusion $\times$ 5 days), then weekly interferon alfa (9 million U SC 3 $\times$ weekly)
- Combination therapy: 5-FU (450 mg/m^2 IV daily $\times$ 5 days). At 28 days, begin 5-FU (450 mg/m^2 IV weekly $\times$ 48 weeks) + levamisole (50 mg PO q8h $\times$ 6 days), every 2 weeks starting day 1 for 1 year
- For liver metastasis: hepatic artery continuous infusion of heparin (5000 U/day) with 5-FU (800 mg/m^2 IV daily $\times$ 4 days, then 600 mg/m^2 for a maximum of 17 days, as tolerated). For an implanted pump: floxuridine (0.1–0.15 mg/kg/day) in heparinized saline (200 U/ml) $\times$ 2 weeks

Potential Problems
- Anorexia
- Anxiety
- Changes in body image
- Colostomy
- Dehydration
- Electrolyte imbalances
- Infection
- Periostomal skin breakdown
- Stomatitis
- Weight loss

Potential Oncologic Emergencies
- Bowel obstruction
- Septic shock
- SIADH

Prognosis
- Using AJCC/UICC system, 5-year survival: Stage I, 85–90%; Stage II, 65–75%; Stage III, 55%; Stage IV, < 5%

Cutaneous T-Cell Lymphoma

Epidemiology

- Annual incidence 0.4 cases per 100,000
- Average age at presentation 50–60 years
- Also known as *mycosis fungoides*

Etiology/Risk Factors

- None known

Signs and Symptoms

- Alopecia
- Cutaneous skin lesions
- Nail dystrophy
- Peripheral lymphadenopathy
- Pruritus

Diagnostic Tests

- Bone marrow biopsy
- CBC
- Chest and abdominal CT
- Chest radiography
- Liver biopsy
- Liver function tests
- Lymph node biopsy
- Serum chemistries
- Sézary cell count
- Skin biopsy
- Whole-body mapping of skin lesions

Metastatic Sites

- Liver
- Lung
- Lymph nodes

Treatment

- Current initial therapies are tailored to extent of the disease, total tumor burden, and type of disease present
- Therapeutic options for cutaneous T-cell lymphoma:
  - Topical therapy: corticosteroids, nitrogen mustard, BCNU
  - Ultraviolet B phototherapy
  - PUVA photochemotherapy
  - Radiotherapy with electron beam
  - Systemic chemotherapy with single agents (e.g., methotrexate, cisplatin, etoposide, bleomycin, doxorubicin, vincristine, or vinblastine) or combination regimens (e.g., cyclophosphamide, vincristine, prednisone, doxorubicin, methotrexate)
  - Combined-modality therapy
  - Extracorporeal photochemotherapy
  - Interferons
  - Monoclonal antibody therapy
  - Retinoids
  - Purine nucleoside analogues (e.g., 2´-deoxycoformycin, fludarabine, 2-chloro-2´-deoxyadenosine)
  - Cyclosporine
  - Acyclovir
  - Thymopentin
  - Autologous BMT

Potential Problems

- Body image disturbance
- Infection
- Pain
- Pruritus

Potential Oncologic Emergencies

- Septic shock

Prognosis

- In one series, the 5-year survival rates were as follows: Stage I, 80–90%; Stage II, 60–70%; Stage IIB, 30%; Stage III 40–50%; Stage IV, 25–35%

Endometrial Cancer

Epidemiology
- 95% of all cancers of the uterus
- Adenocarcinomas arise from the endometrium
- Average age at presentation, 59 years
- Incidence is higher in white women, as compared with blacks

Etiology/Risk Factors
- Length of menstruation > 7 days
- Menarche before age 12 years
- Nulliparity
- Obesity
- Use of estrogen
- Use of tamoxifen

Signs and Symptoms
- Abnormal vaginal bleeding
- Pelvic mass
- Pelvic pain
- Pyometra

Diagnostic Tests
- Abdominal and pelvic CT
- Barium enema
- Blood glucose
- CA-125
- CBC
- Chest radiography
- Colonoscopy
- Creatinine
- Endometrial biopsy
- Fractional D & C
- Liver function tests
- MRI
- PAP smear
- Pelvic examination
- Rectal examination
- Serum electrolytes
- Total bilirubin level
- Vaginal probe ultrasonography

Metastatic Sites
- Abdomen
- Bone
- Brain
- Lung

Treatment
- Hysterectomy, bilateral salpingo-oophorectomy, and pelvic and paraaortic lymph node sampling is the treatment of choice for Stage I disease
- Radiation therapy with 5000 cGy to the whole pelvis is often recommended for more than superficial invasion, advanced-grade disease, or positive nodes
- Metastatic disease may require a combination of surgery, radiation therapy, and chemotherapy
- Chemotherapy drugs commonly used include cisplatin, doxorubicin, and cyclophosphamide

Potential Problems
- Altered urinary elimination
- Body image disturbance
- Nutritional deficit
- Pain

Potential Oncologic Emergencies
- Intestinal obstruction
- Spinal cord compression
- Third-space syndrome

Prognosis
- Several factors influence prognosis, including patient's age, histology of the tumor, depth of myometrial invasion, peritoneal invasion, and presence of distant metastases

Esophageal Cancer: Adenocarcinoma

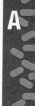

Epidemiology

- Usually occurs in the lower third of the esophagus
- Incidence is increasing
- Occurs in fifth or sixth decade of life

Etiology/Risk Factors

- Barrett's esophagus
- Gastroesophageal reflux
- Impaired host defenses

Signs and Symptoms

- Chronic antacid use
- Dysphagia
- Heartburn
- Odynophagia
- Weight loss

Diagnostic Tests

- Barium esophagram
- Bone scan
- CT of abdomen
- CT chest
- Endoscopy and biopsy
- Transesophageal endoscopic ultrasonography

Metastatic Sites

- Adrenal glands
- Bone
- Celiac axis
- Liver
- Lymph nodes
- Pericardium
- Trachea

Treatment

- Endoscopic procedures (i.e., esophageal intubation, laser therapy, electrofulguration, brachytherapy) are used to restore patency of the esophagus
- Surgery can be used as a single modality with a partial esophagogastrectomy being performed
- Chemotherapy is used as a single therapy or as part of a multimodal regimen; most active drugs are cisplatin and mitomycin; promising agents include vindesine, venorelbine, methyl-GAG, and paclitaxel
- Radiation therapy as a single modality is used for cure and palliation
- Multimodal therapy sequences that have been used include surgery with pre- or postoperative radiation therapy; surgery following preoperative chemotherapy; surgery following concomitant chemotherapy and radiation therapy; and chemotherapy and radiation therapy

Potential Problems

- Anorexia
- Decreased nutritional intake
- Esophagitis
- Fatigue
- Fever
- Gastroesophageal reflux
- Ineffective airway clearance
- Nausea and vomiting
- Pain

Potential Oncologic Emergencies

- Acute airway obstruction
- Pleural effusions
- Pneumonia

Prognosis

- Median survival 12–29 months

Esophageal Cancer: Squamous Cell Carcinoma

Epidemiology
- Usually occurs in the middle third of the esophagus
- Most common histologic type of esophageal cancer
- Occurs in sixth to seventh decade of life

Etiology/Risk Factors
- Chronic esophageal irritation
- Tobacco use
- Alcohol consumption
- High-starch diet
- Achalasia
- Lye ingestion
- Radiation therapy
- Plummer-Vinson syndrome
- History of head and neck cancer
- Impaired host defenses

Signs and Symptoms
- Difficulty swallowing
- Epigastric pain
- Hoarseness
- Horner's syndrome
- Odynophagia
- Substernal pain
- Supraclavicular adenopathy
- Tracheoesophageal fistula
- Weight loss

Diagnostic Tests
- Barium esophagram
- Bone scan
- Bronchoscope
- CT of abdomen
- CT of chest
- Endoscopy and biopsy
- Transesophageal endoscopic ultrasonography

Metastatic Sites
- Adrenal glands
- Bone
- Celiac axis
- Liver
- Lymph nodes
- Pericardium
- Trachea

Treatment
- Endoscopic procedures (i.e., esophageal intubation, laser therapy, electrofulguration, brachytherapy) are used to restore esophageal patency
- Surgery (partial esophagogastrectomy) can be used as a single modality
- Chemotherapy is used as a single therapy or as part of a multimodal regimen; most active drugs are cisplatin and mitomycin; promising agents include vindesine, venorelbine, methyl-GAG, and paclitaxel
- Radiation therapy as a single modality is used for cure and palliation
- Multimodal therapy sequences that have been used include surgery with pre- or postoperative radiation therapy; surgery following preoperative chemotherapy; surgery following concomitant chemotherapy and radiation therapy; and chemotherapy and radiation therapy

Potential Problems
- Anorexia
- Decreased nutritional intake
- Esophagitis
- Fatigue
- Fever
- Gastroesophageal reflux
- Ineffective airway clearance
- Nausea and vomiting
- Pain

Potential Oncologic Emergencies
- Acute airway obstruction
- Pleural effusions
- Pneumonia

Prognosis
- Median survival 12–29 months

Cancer in the Floor of the Mouth

Epidemiology
- Approximately 11,000 new cases per year
- Approximately 2300 deaths per year

Etiology/Risk Factors
- Tobacco use
- Alcohol consumption

Signs and Symptoms
- Aspiration symptoms
- Deep-seated ear pain
- Dysphagia
- Easy bleeding of the mucosal surface
- Erythroplakia
- Leukoplakia
- Neck mass
- Repeated bleeding from the oral cavity
- Slow-healing sore
- Unilateral pain

Diagnostic Tests
- Biopsy
- Bone scan
- CBC
- CT
- Chest radiography
- Complete head and neck exam
- Dental consult
- Panendoscopy
- Serum chemistries
- Videoendoscopic exam

Metastatic Sites
- Bone
- Brain
- Liver
- Lung
- Regional lymph nodes

Treatment
- Surgery and radiation therapy are equally effective in treating early-stage (T1 or T2) tumors of the floor of the mouth
- Laser surgery decreases pain and reduces scarring and swelling
- Patients with tumors that involve the mandible usually require partial mandibulectomy and neck dissection

Potential Problems
- Altered sense of smell
- Anorexia
- Anxiety
- Body image disturbance
- Decreased nutritional intake
- Dental problems
- Dysphagia
- Grieving
- Impaired verbal communication
- Ineffective breathing pattern
- Pain
- Stomatitis
- Taste changes
- Xerostomia

Potential Oncologic Emergencies
- Airway obstruction
- Carotid hemorrhage
- Pneumonia

Prognosis
- For Stage I tumors, survival rates range from 80–90%; for Stage III disease, 5-year survival ranges from 25–66%

Gallbladder Cancer

Epidemiology
- 6000 new cases per year
- Peak incidence in persons aged 50–70 years
- Female-male ratio 3:1

Etiology
- Exact cause is unknown
- Mostly associated with gallstones but no evidence of cause-and-effect relationship
- Increased incidence in patients with an anomalous pancreaticobiliary union
- Higher rate in younger native Americans from Southwest

Signs and Symptoms
- Anorexia
- Ascites
- Chills and fever
- Fatty-food intolerance
- Jaundice
- Malaise
- Nausea, vomiting
- Palpable gallbaldder
- Steady and gnawing pain and tenderness
- Weight loss

Diagnostic Tests
- Alkaline phosphatase
- Bilirubin
- CBC
- CT
- ERCP
- Hepatic transaminase
- PTC
- Ultrasonography

Metastatic Sites
- Bone
- Duodenum or transverse colon
- Extrahepatic bile ducts
- Gallbladder fossa of the liver
- Liver
- Lung
- Pancreas
- Paraaortic nodes
- Portal vein or hepatic artery
- Regional cystic, choledochal, or pancreaticoduodenal nodes

Treatment

- Surgery
  - Standard surgery (cholecystectomy)
  - Radical procedures, including the gallbladder fossa of the liver, regional nodes, and the gallbladder for advanced-stage disease (Stage 3)
  - Palliative surgery
- Radiation therapy
  - External-beam radiotherapy (total dose 4000–5000 cGy)
  - Intraoperative radiotherapy
  - Intracavitary radiotherapy
  - Preoperative and/or postoperative radiation
  - Palliative therapy for relief of jaundice and osseous pain
- Chemotherapy
  - Single agent: 5-FU (500 mg/m^2 IV on days 1–5 every 4 weeks or 500–600 mg/m^2 IV weekly)
  - Combination chemotherapy: FAM: 5-FU (600 mg/m^2 IV on days 1, 8, 29, 36), doxorubicin (30 mg/m^2 IV on days 1 and 29), and mitomycin (10 mg/m^2 IV on day 1). Repeat every 8 weeks.
- Nonsurgical management
  - Percutaneous or endoscopic biliary decompression

Potential Problems
- Anorexia
- Anxiety
- Continuing percutaneous biliary decompression
- Diarrhea
- Fatty-food intolerance
- Infection
- Melena

Potential Oncologic Emergencies
- Common bile duct obstruction
- Septic shock

Prognosis
- Overall survival rate < 5% (average survival after diagnosis is about 9 months)
- 5-year survival rates: Stage III, 15%; Stage IV, < 1%

Glioblastoma

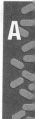

Epidemiology

- Approximately 2740 cases per year
- Most common brain tumor
- Small peak in childhood; maximum peak between age 60 and 80 years

Etiology/Risk Factors

- Unknown
- Genetic defect

Signs and Symptoms

- General manifestations
  - Headache
  - Mental status changes
  - Papilledema
  - Pupillary changes
  - Seizures
  - Vasomotor and autonomic changes
  - Vomiting
- Focal manifestations depend on the location of the tumor
  - Changes in cognitive functioning
  - Gait disturbance
  - Hearing impairment
  - Meningeal signs
  - Neuroendocrine disturbances
  - Paresthesias
  - Personality changes
  - Visual changes

Diagnostic Tests

- Biopsy
- CT
- PET
- MRI

Metastatic Sites

- None

Treatment

- Cytoreduction is accomplished with multimodal treatment
- Surgery: extent of surgery depends on location of the tumor; extends survival in low-grade gliomas
- Radiation therapy: most important single modality in high-grade gliomas; minimum dose is 60 Gy to the tumor
- Chemotherapy: limited value; best drugs are BCNU, CCNU, procarbazine, and vincristine

Potential Problems

- Bradycardia
- Decreased mobility
- Impaired cognition
- Ineffective breathing pattern
- Mood disturbance
- Nausea and vomiting
- Pain
- Potential for injury
- Self-care deficit
- Sensory-perceptual deficit

Potential Oncologic Emergencies

- Brain stem herniation
- Increased intracranial pressure
- Respiratory arrest

Prognosis

- Median survival 10–12 months; 2-year survival 10%

Glioma

Epidemiology
- Occurs mostly in children
- Occurs in the brain stem

Etiology/Risk Factors
- Neurofibromatosis
- Genetic defect

Signs and Symptoms
- Ataxia
- Cranial nerve dysfunction
- Headache
- Hemiplegia
- Hemianesthesia
- Intention tremor
- Mental status changes
- Nystagmus

Diagnostic Tests
- CT
- MRI
- Stereotactic biopsy

Metastatic Sites
- None

Treatment
- Surgical resection of tumor is rarely possible
- Radiation therapy is the mainstay of treatment

Potential Problems
- Anxiety
- Decreased mobility
- Fear
- Nausea and vomiting
- Pain
- Potential for injury

Potential Oncologic Emergencies
- Brain stem herniation
- Increased intracranial pressure
- Respiratory arrest

Prognosis
- Extremely poor

Head and Neck Cancer

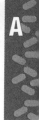

Epidemiology

- Represents approximately 5% of all malignancies
- More common in males
- More common in blacks and Asians
- Peak incidence at age 50

Etiology/Risk Factors

- Tobacco use
- Alcohol consumption

Signs and Symptoms

- Aspiration symptoms
- Deep-seated ear pain
- Dysphagia
- Easy bleeding of the mucosal surface
- Erythroplakia
- Leukoplakia
- Neck mass
- Repeated bleeding from the nose or oral cavity
- Slow-healing sore
- Unilateral pain

Diagnostic Tests

- Biopsy
- Bone scan
- CBC
- CT
- Chest radiography
- Complete head and neck exam
- Dental consult
- Panendoscopy
- Serum chemistries
- Videoendoscopic exam

Metastatic Sites

- Bone
- Brain
- Liver
- Lung
- Regional lymph nodes

Treatment

- Major source of treatment failure is local and regional recurrence
- Multidisciplinary management is necessary and usually involves a surgeon, radiation and medical oncologists, and rehabilitation personnel
- Surgery is extremely complex, and the nature of the procedure is determined by the size and location of the tumor
- Radiation may be used alone (for early-stage lesions) or in combination with surgery
- Chemotherapy may be used as a palliative treatment for recurrent or metastatic disease. A common regimen combines cisplatin with 5-FU

Potential Problems

- Altered sense of smell
- Anorexia
- Anxiety
- Body image disturbance
- Decreased nutritional intake
- Dental problems
- Dysphagia
- Fatigue
- Grieving
- Impaired verbal communication
- Ineffective breathing pattern
- Pain
- Stomatitis
- Taste changes
- Xerostomia

Potential Oncologic Emergencies

- Airway obstruction
- Carotid hemorrhage
- Pneumonia

Prognosis

- Overall cure rate for head and neck cancer < 50%

Hepatocellular Cancer

Epidemiology
- One of the 10 most common human cancers
- One million new cases per year, worldwide

Etiology/Risk Factors
- Cirrhosis
- Chronic hepatitis B infection
- Hepatitis C infection
- Chemical exposure: aflatoxins B1 and G; nitrosamines
- Gender: 6–10 times more prevalent in males than in females

Signs and Symptoms
- Abdominal pain and swelling
- Anorexia
- Ascites
- Esophageal varices
- Fever
- Hematemesis
- Hepatomegaly
- Jaundice
- Splenomegaly
- Vomiting
- Weakness
- Weight loss

Diagnostic Tests
- Abdominal CT
- Abdominal ultrasound
- Coagulation profile
- Liver biopsy
- Liver enzymes
- MRI
- Serum α-fetoprotein

Metastatic Sites
- Adrenal glands
- Bile ducts
- Bone
- Lung
- Peritoneal surfaces
- Regional lymph nodes

Treatment
- Complete surgical resection provides the best opportunity for long-term survival
- Systemic chemotherapy primarily palliative; most common agent used is 5-FU
- Intraarterial chemotherapy with fluorodeoxyuridine has been tried
- Hepatic artery chemoembolization, alone or in combination with intraarterial chemotherapy, has been used

Potential Problems
- Altered level of consciousness
- Ascites
- Fluid volume deficit
- Impaired mobility
- Impaired skin integrity
- Nutritional deficit
- Pain
- Pruritus

Potential Oncologic Emergencies
- Disseminated intravascular coagulation
- Erythrocytosis
- Hypercalcemia
- Hypoglycemia

Prognosis
- Prognosis is variable, depending on extent of the disease and size of tumor at diagnosis

Hodgkin's Disease

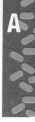

Epidemiology
- About 8000 cases per year in the United States
- Bimodal age distribution; peaks at ages 20–24 years and 80–84 years
- Increased incidence in HIV-positive persons

Etiology/Risk Factors
- Etiology is unknown
- Associated with ataxia telangiectasia

Signs and Symptoms
- Abdominal mass
- Bone pain
- Elevated ESR
- Fever
- Leukocytosis
- Lymph node enlargement
- Mediastinal mass
- Night sweats
- Pruritus
- Splenomegaly
- Thrombocytopenia
- Weight loss

Diagnostic Tests
- Abdominal CT
- Bipedal lymphangiography
- Bone marrow biopsy
- BUN and creatinine levels
- CBC
- Chest CT
- Chest radiography
- Echocardiogram
- ESR
- Gallium scan
- Laparotomy
- Liver biopsy
- Liver function tests
- Lymph node biopsy
- MRI
- Physical examination
- Serum alkaline phosphatase
- Technetium bone scan
- Ultrasonography

Metastatic Sites
- Bone
- Liver
- Lung

Treatment
- Primary treatment determined by stage of disease: total nodal or subtotal nodal radiation therapy for early-stage disease; combination chemotherapy for advanced-stage disease; combined multimodal therapy for massive mediastinal disease

Potential Problems
- Fatigue
- Infection
- Mucositis
- Nutritional deficit
- Pain

Potential Oncologic Emergencies
- Neoplastic cardiac tamponade
- Septic shock

Prognosis
- Cure rate is 75–80% with appropriate treatment

Kidney Cancer: Renal Cell Carcinoma

Epidemiology
- Approximately 29,000 new cases per year
- Approximately 85% of cancers of the kidney are renal cell
- Accounts for 2% of all cancers in adults
- Male-female ratio approximately 2:1

Etiology/Risk Factors
- High-fat diet
- Obesity
- Tobacco use
- von Hippel-Lindau disease

Signs and Symptoms
- Early: hematuria, flank pain, palpable renal mass
- Late: nonspecific symptoms such as fever, weight loss, nausea, fatigue; anemia; paraneoplastic syndromes (including hypercalcemia, polycythemia, hypertension); hepatic dysfunction; cardiac failure; varicocele; pain

Diagnostic Tests
- Blood chemistries
- CBC
- Chest radiography
- CT and/or MRI
- Radionuclide bone scan (for patients with bone pain)
- Ultrasonography

Metastatic Sites
- Adrenal gland
- Bone
- Brain
- Contralateral kidney
- Liver
- Lungs

Treatment

- Surgery: radical nephrectomy, frequently with lymphadenectomy, is potentially curative treatment for localized disease (Stages I–III); partial nephrectomy is an option when preservation of functional renal parenchyma is important (e.g., bilateral disease)
- Immunotherapy (biologic response–modifier therapy): for advanced disease
  - IL-2 by intravenous bolus or continuous infusion
  - IFN: IFN-alfa has been best studied; 5–10 million U/day administered at least 3 times per week
- Radiation therapy for palliative treatment of bone metastases or inoperable tumor
- Chemotherapy: vinblastine (5–6 mg/m^2 IV weekly) or lomustine (130 mg/m^2 PO, every 6 weeks)
- Renal artery embolization may be used for tumor reduction of very large masses or for palliative treatment of pain and hematuria due to inoperable tumors
- Hormone therapy: megestrol acetate (160 mg PO daily) or tamoxifen (10 mg PO b.i.d.) or medroxyprogesterone (800 mg IM weekly)

Potential Problems
- Abnormal liver function tests
- Anorexia
- Cardiac toxicity
- Chills
- Diarrhea
- Fatigue
- Fever
- Flulike symptoms
- Hyperbilirubinemia
- Hypotension
- Lethargy
- Leukopenia
- Malaise
- Myalgia
- Nausea and vomiting
- Neurologic abnormalities
- Occasional dyspnea
- Oliguria
- Pain
- Pruritus
- Rash
- Thrombocytopenia
- Vascular/capillary leak syndrome
- Weight gain
- Weight loss

Potential Oncologic Emergencies
- GI obstruction
- Hypercalcemia
- Spinal cord compression

Prognosis
- 5-year survival with treatment (using staging system of Robson, Churchill, and Anderson): Stage I, 70%; Stage II, 50%; Stage III, 35%; Stage IV, 5%

Laryngeal Cancer

Epidemiology

- Approximately 11,600 new cases per year
- Approximately 4090 deaths per year
- Most tumors involve the supraglottic and glottic levels

Etiology/Risk Factors

- Tobacco use
- Alcohol consumption
- Carotene deficiency
- Asbestos exposure

Signs and Symptoms

- Aspiration symptoms
- Deep-seated ear pain
- Dysphagia
- Hoarseness
- Neck mass
- Slow-healing sore
- Unilateral pain

Diagnostic Tests

- Biopsy
- Bone scan
- CBC
- CT
- Chest radiography
- Complete head and neck exam
- Dental consult
- Panendoscopy
- Serum chemistries
- Videoendoscopic exam

Metastatic Sites

- Bone
- Brain
- Liver
- Lung
- Regional lymph nodes

Treatment

- Approach to treatment is based on the stage of the disease and whether the tumor lies in the glottic or supraglottic area
- Early stage disease (T1, N0) is usually treated with radiation therapy or a supraglottic laryngectomy
- Advanced-stage disease is treated with a total laryngectomy and postoperative radiation therapy or induction chemotherapy, radiation therapy, and surgery (i.e., total laryngectomy)

Potential Problems

- Altered sense of smell
- Anorexia
- Anxiety
- Body image disturbance
- Decreased nutritional intake
- Dental problems
- Dysphagia
- Grieving
- Impaired verbal communication
- Ineffective breathing pattern
- Pain
- Stomatitis
- Taste changes
- Xerostomia

Potential Oncologic Emergencies

- Airway obstruction
- Carotid hemorrhage
- Pneumonia

Prognosis

- Overall 5-year survival 23–83%, depending on the stage of the disease

Leukemia: Acute Lymphoblastic

Epidemiology
- Approximately 4200 new cases per year
- Biologically and clinically heterogeneous group of diseases

Etiology/Risk Factors
- Inherited conditions
  - Chromosome breakage disorders
  - Immunodeficiency
  - Chromosome disorders
  - Familial predisposition
- Viruses
- Environmental factors
  - Radiation
  - Hair dyes
  - Tobacco
  - Farming

Signs and Symptoms
- Anemia
- Chest pain
- Chills
- Ecchymosis
- Elevated LDH
- Epistaxis
- Fatigue
- Fever
- Hepatosplenomegaly
- Hyperuricemia
- Malaise
- Neutropenia
- Pallor
- Petechiae
- Tachycardia
- Thrombocytopenia
- Weakness

Diagnostic Tests
- Blood type
- Bone marrow biopsy
- Cardiac ejection fraction
- CBC with differential
- Chemistry profile
- Chest radiography
- Coagulation profile
- Cytomegalovius cytology
- ECG
- History and physical exam
- HLA type
- Lumbar puncture

Metastatic Sites
- CNS

Treatment

- Remission induction therapy: vincristine, prednisone, and daunorubicin (VPD) are the most common agents used for induction; a number of variations of VPD exist; options are shown in brackets
  - VPD: Vincristine (2 mg IV on days 1, 8, 15, [22]) and prednisone (40 or 60 mg/m^2 PO on days 1–28 to 1–35, followed by a rapid taper) and daunorubicin (45 mg/m^2 IV on days 1–3); L-asparaginase (500 IU/kg IV on days 22–32)
  - DVPL: daunorubicin (60 mg/m^2 IV on days 1–3); vincristine (2 mg IV on days 1, 8, 15, 22); prednisone (60 mg/m^2 PO on days 1–28); and L-asparaginase (6000 U/m^2 IM on days 17–28)
- Remission induction therapy in patients with impaired cardiac function: methotrexate (100 mg/m^2 IV on day 1); vincristine (2 mg IV on day 2); L-asparaginase (500 IU/kg IV infusion on day 2); and dexamethasone (6 mg/m^2 PO on days 1–10) (MOAD regimen)
- CNS prophylaxis: cranial irradiation (18 to 24 Gy in 2-Gy fractions) with intrathecal methotrexate (12 mg/m^2 once a week for 6 weeks)
- Consolidation therapy (two courses): cytarabine (75 mg/m^2 SC on days 1–4 and 8–11); 6-mercaptopurine (60 mg/m^2 PO on days 1–14); L-asparaginase (6000 IU/m^2 IM on days 15, 18, 22, 25); and vincristine (2 mg IV on days 15 and 22)
- Maintenance therapy (for 102 weeks, 28-day cycles): 6-mercaptopurine (60 mg/m^2 PO daily); methotrexate (20 mg/m^2 PO weekly); prednisone (60 mg/m^2 PO on days 1–5); and vincristine (7 mg IV on day 1)
- Bone marrow transplantation

Potential Problems
- Alopecia
- Body image disturbance
- Depression
- Fatigue
- Fluid volume deficit
- High risk for injury
- Infection
- Mucositis
- Nutritional deficit
- Sleep pattern disturbance

Potential Oncologic Emergencies
- DIC
- Septic shock
- Tumor lysis syndrome

Prognosis
- Numerous factors influence whether or not an individual achieves a complete response as well as the duration of survival: age, WBC count, cytogenetic abnormalities, time to response, and immunophenotype

Leukemia: Acute Nonlymphocytic

Epidemiology

- Myeloblasts, promyelocytes, monoblasts, promonocytes, megakaryocytes make up more than 30% of the nucleated marrow cells
- Three cases per 100,000 annually

Etiology/Risk Factors

- Increasing age
- Occupational exposure to chemicals (e.g., benzene)
- Inherited genetic disorders (e.g., Bloom's syndrome, Fanconi's anemia, Down's syndrome)
- Chemotherapeutic agents (e.g., cyclophosphamide, chlorambucil, etoposide, teniposide)
- Radiation exposure
- History of bone marrow disease

Signs and Symptoms

- Anemia
- Chest pain
- Chills
- Ecchymosis
- Elevated LDH
- Epistaxis
- Fatigue
- Fever
- Hepatosplenomegaly
- Hyperuricemia
- Malaise
- Neutropenia
- Pallor
- Petechiae
- Tachycardia
- Thrombocytopenia
- Weakness

Diagnostic Tests

- Blood type
- Bone marrow biopsy
- Cardiac ejection fraction
- CBC with differential
- Chemistry profile
- Chest radiography
- Coagulation profile
- CMV cytology
- ECG
- History and physical exam
- HLA type
- Karyotyping
- Lumbar puncture

Metastatic Sites

- CNS

Treatment

- Remission induction therapy: the two most common programs are "7 + 3" and "DAT."
  - "7 + 3" combination: cytarabine (100 mg/m^2 per day in continuous IV infusion on days 1 and 7) + daunorubicin (45 mg/m^2 IV push on days 1 and 3)
  - DAT regimen: cytarabine (25 mg/m^2 IV push, followed by 200 mg/m^2 per day in continuous infusion on days 1 and 5) and daunorubicin (60 mg/m^2 IV push on days 1 and 3) + thioguanine (100 mg/m^2 PO every 12 hours, on days 1–5)
- Maintenance therapy can involve a variety of therapeutic regimens
- Bone marrow transplantation

Potential Problems

- Alopecia
- Body image disturbance
- Fatigue
- Fluid volume deficit
- High risk for injury
- Infection
- Mucositis
- Nutritional deficit
- Sleep pattern disturbance

Potential Oncologic Emergencies

- Disseminated intravascular coagulation
- Septic shock
- Tumor lysis syndrome

Prognosis

- In general, remission duration is 12–15 months and overall survival is 18–24 months with maintenance chemotherapy

Leukemia: Chronic Lymphocytic

Epidemiology

- 11,000 new cases per year
- Male-female ratio 2:1
- Median age is 60 years

Etiology/Risk Factors

- No known retroviral association
- Slightly increased incidence following radiation exposure in the Japanese bombings
- Risk factors unknown

Signs and Symptoms

- Early: nonspecific complaints such as fatigue or malaise; possible varying degrees of lymphadenopathy, hepatomegaly, or splenomegaly
- Late: anemia, lymphadenopathy, infections, and/or complications to the intestinal mucosa, lungs, skin, or bone

Diagnostic Tests

- Bone scan
- Bone marrow aspiration
- BUN
- CBC
- Chest radiography
- Coagulation profile
- Creatinine
- CT
- Electrolyte panel
- Liver function tests
- Lumbar puncture
- MRI
- Serum uric acid levels

Sites of Metastasis

- May diffusely involve all organs. Local infiltration to liver, lung, GI tract, skin, kidneys, lymph nodes, CNS, and spleen

Treatment

- An initial observational period of 3 to 6 months may be indicated to ascertain the course of the disease
- Chemotherapy:
  - Chlorambucil (0.2 mg/kg daily; 0.4–1.0 mg/kg every 4 weeks; or 0.4–0.6 mg/kg every 4–6 weeks) + prednisone (60–100 mg/m^2)
  - Fludarabine (25 mg/m^2 per day for 5 days every 4 weeks)
  - High-dose prednisone (0.5–1.0 mg/kg per day)
- Surgery: possible splenectomy
- Biotherapy:
  - Immunoglobulin infusion (400 mg/kg every 3 weeks) for patients with a history of one or more major infections or with low IgG levels
  - IFN-α (5 million U/m^2 SC per day)
- Radiation:
  - Local radiation is given for lymphadenopathy that compromises vital organ function or bone pain relief (0.05–0.10 Gy/day 3–4 times a week to a total dose of 1000–4000 cGy)
  - Total body radiation (400 cGy in 5- to 10-cGy daily fractions)
  - Splenic radiation given for painful splenomegaly, progressive lymphocytosis, anemia, or thrombocytopenia (1200–1500 cGy in 25–50 cGy fractions over 2–3 weeks)
- Autogenic and allogenic BMT: too early to determine the results of BMT

Patient Problems

- Anemia
- Anorexia
- Dehydration
- Fatigue
- Infection
- Pain
- Thrombocytopenia
- Weight loss

Potential Oncologic Emergencies

- Septic shock
- Spinal cord compression

Prognosis

- Using the International Workshop on CLL Staging System, median survival in years: Stage A, > 9; Stage B, 5; Stage C, 2

Leukemia: Chronic Myelogenous

Epidemiology

- More than 600,000 cases per year in the United States
- Accounts for 15–20% of all leukemias
- Peaks in fifth to sixth decades
- Slight male predominance

Etiology/Risk Factors

- Radiation exposure
- Occupational exposure to benzene

Signs and Symptoms

- Abdominal fullness
- Anemia
- Bone pain
- Fatigue
- Fever
- Leukocytosis
- Malaise
- Night sweats
- Splenomegaly
- Weight loss

Diagnostic Tests

- Bone marrow biopsy
- CBC
- Cytogenic analysis
- Presence of the Philadelphia chromosome
- Serum B_{12} level
- Serum uric acid level
- WBC count with differential

Metastatic Site

- CNS

Treatment

- Busulfan is given to initially lower WBC count in doses of 2.0 mg/m^2 (i.e., 4 mg PO per day) or 4.0 mg/m^2 (i.e., 8 mg PO per day) until the counts reach 15,000–20,000/μl
- Hydroxyurea: recommended initial dose is 0.5–1.5 g/m^2 PO per day until the counts reach 10,000–15,000/μl
- Allogeneic BMT recommended for young patients if an HLA-identical sibling is available
- Interferon-α: administered SC daily in a dose of 5×10^6 U

Potential Problems

- Depression
- Fatigue
- Fluid volume deficit
- High risk for injury
- Infection
- Nutritional deficit
- Pain

Potential Oncologic Emergencies

- DIC
- Septic shock
- Tumor lysis syndrome

Prognosis

- Prognosis is extremely poor at the time of blast crisis; only 25% of patients survive therapy

Leukemia: Hairy Cell

Epidemiology
- 2% of the leukemias in the United States
- 600 new cases per year
- Characterized by circulating B lymphocytes that display prominent cytoplasmic projections
- Patients tend to be elderly

Etiology/Risk Factors
- Cause is unknown
- Disease of middle-aged men
- Male-female ratio is 4:1
- Jewish descent

Signs and Symptoms
- Anemia
- Ecchymosis
- Fatigue
- Hepatomegaly
- Infection
- Lymphadenopathy
- Neutropenia
- Petechiae
- Splenomegaly
- Thrombocytopenia
- Weakness

Diagnostic Tests
- Bone marrow biopsy
- CT
- History and physical examination
- Immunophenotypic analysis of the peripheral blood or bone marrow
- Review of peripheral blood smear
- Tartrate-resistant acid phosphatase staining of the peripheral blood or buffy coat

Metastatic Sites
- Skeleton

Treatment

- 10% of patients with hairy cell leukemia may never require treatment
- Splenectomy: first standard therapy, now has a diminished role owing to other more effective therapies
- IFN-α: standard dose is 2 million U/m^2 SC three times a week for 12 months
- 2'-Deoxycoformycin: recommended dose is 4 mg/m^2 IV every other week for 3–6 months
- 2-Chloro-2'-deoxyadenosine: single 7-day course at 0.1 mg/kg/day by continuous IV infusion

Potential Problems
- Fatigue
- Fever
- Flulike syndrome
- Infection
- Myalgias
- Nausea and vomiting
- Nutritional deficit
- Photosensitivity

Potential Oncologic Emergencies
- DIC
- Pleural effusions
- *Pneumocystis carinii* pneumonia
- Septic shock

Prognosis
- Complete response rates are as follows: 10% with IFN-α; 64% with 2'-deoxycoformycin; 84% with 2-chloro-2'-deoxyadenosine

Lung Cancer: Non–Small Cell

Epidemiology

- 75–80% of all lung cancer
- More common in men (black men > white men)
- Incidence in women rising
- Age 50–70 years
- Types: squamous cell (25–30%); adenocarcinoma (25–30%); large cell (10–20%)

Etiology/Risk Factors

- Low intake of beta-carotene
- Exposure to radon, asbestos, other carcinogens
- Positive family history
- Chronic obstructive pulmonary disease
- Smoking/passive smoking

Signs and Symptoms

- Early: none or nonspecific
- Late: persistent cough, dyspnea, change in breathing pattern, anorexia, weight loss, weakness, hemoptysis, dysphagia, clubbing, chest pain, hoarseness, wheezing, stridor, Horner's syndrome

Diagnostic Tests

- Bronchoscopy
- Chest CT
- Chest radiography
- Lymph node biopsy
- Mediastinoscopy
- Sputum cytology

Metastatic Sites

- Bone
- Bone marrow
- Brain
- Liver
- Lymph nodes

Treatment

- Surgery: standard treatment for patients with Stage I or II disease
- Radiation: adjuvant therapy for Stage II disease; standard treatment for unresectable Stage IIIa and IIIb disease
- Chemotherapy: adjuvant therapy for Stage II, IIIa, or IIIb disease; primary treatment for Stage IV disease
  - CAP: cyclophosphamide (400 mg/m^2 IV) + adriamycin (40 mg/m^2 IV) + cisplatin (40 mg/m^2 IV); repeat every 4 weeks
  - VP: vindesine (3 mg/m^2 IV weekly × 4, then every 2 weeks) + cisplatin (120 mg/m^2 IV on days 1 and 29, then every 6 weeks)

Potential Problems

- Dysphagia
- Electrolyte imbalance
- Flulike symptoms
- Infection
- Weakness
- Weight loss

Potential Oncologic Emergencies

- Hypercalcemia
- Superior vena cava syndrome
- SIADH

Prognosis

- Using AJCC systems, 5-year survival: Stage I, 45%; Stage II, 25%; Stage IIIa, 15%; Stage IIIb, < 5%; Stage IV, < 1%

Lung Cancer: Small Cell (Oat Cell)

Epidemiology

- 20–25% of all lung cancers
- Males 50–70 years old (black males > white males)
- Incidence in females increasing
- 40,000 deaths annually

Etiology/Risk Factors

- Low dietary intake of beta-carotene
- Exposure to radon, asbestos, arsenic, other carcinogens
- Positive family history
- Smoking/secondary smoke

Signs and Symptoms

- Early: none or nonspecific
- Late: persistent cough, change in breathing habits, hemoptysis, hoarseness, weight loss, weakness, anorexia, clubbing, Horner's syndrome, wheezing, recurrent lung infection, bone pain, abdominal pain, chest pain

Diagnostic Tests

- Bone scan
- Bronchoscopy
- Chest CT
- Chest radiography
- Liver function tests
- Lymph node biopsy
- Mediastinoscopy
- Sputum cytology

Metastatic Sites

- Bone
- Bone marrow
- Brain
- Liver

Treatment

- Surgery is an alternative to radiation therapy for limited disease
- Radiation therapy is an adjunct to chemotherapy. Patients may receive whole-brain irradiation (30 Gy in 2 weeks), prophylactically. Chest radiation is given after chemotherapy.
- Chemotherapy: single agents or combination therapy used for remission
  - VAC: vincristine (2 mg IV on day 1) + doxorubicin (50 mg/m^2 IV on day 1) + cyclophosphamide (750 mg/m^2 IV on day 1), repeat every 3 weeks for 4–6 cycles
  - Cisplatin (50 to 80 mg/m^2 IV on day 1) + etoposide (60 mg/m^2 IV on days 1–5 or 100 mg/m^2 on days 1–3), repeat every 3–4 weeks for 4–6 cycles

Potential Problems

- Anxiety
- Cushing's syndrome
- Dyspnea
- Eaton-Lambert syndrome
- Fatigue
- Hypoxemia
- Pain
- Trousseau's syndrome
- Weight loss

Potential Oncologic Emergencies

- Hypercalcemia
- Spinal cord compression
- Superior vena cava syndrome
- SIADH

Prognosis

- Using AJCC systems, 5-year survival is 13% for all stages; 41% for localized stages; 10–25% of patients with limited disease will be alive and disease free in 2 years; < 20% of patients have > 2 years' survival after initiation of chemotherapy

Medulloblastoma

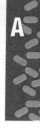

Epidemiology

- Most common primary CNS malignancy in childhood
- Tumor usually occurs in the vermis of the cerebellum
- Peak age is 5 years

Etiology/Risk Factors

- Unknown
- Possible genetic defect

Signs and Symptoms

- Ataxic gait
- Headache
- Intention tremor
- Nausea and vomiting
- Papilledema
- Symptoms of increased intracranial pressure appear early

Diagnostic Tests

- Biopsy
- Bone marrow aspiration
- CSF cytology
- CT
- MRI
- Myelography or spinal MRI with gadolinium contrast

Metastatic Sites

- CSF seeding of the neuraxis
- Bone marrow

Treatment

- Surgery: remove the tumor completely, decompress the cerebral ventricles, and relieve the hydrocephalus
- Craniospinal radiation: required in all patients at a dose of 36 Gy with a boost to the posterior fossa
- Chemotherapy using cyclophosphamide, vincristine, CCNU, and cisplatin in various combinations may increase survival for high-risk patients

Potential Problems

- Impaired cognition
- Impaired mobility
- Nausea and vomiting
- Pain
- Potential for injury

Potential Oncologic Emergencies

- Brain stem herniation
- Increased intracranial pressure
- Respiratory arrest

Prognosis

- 5-year survival among average-risk patients is ≥ 60%

Melanoma

Epidemiology
- 32,000 new cases per year
- 2.6% of all cancers
- Male-female ratio 1.3:1

Etiology/Risk Factors
- Chronic and intermittent exposure to UV radiation
- Dysplastic nevi syndrome
- Exposure to coal tar, pitch, creosote, arsenic, or radium
- Fair complexion, light-colored eyes, light hair
- Family history of melanoma
- Immunosuppression
- Living at lower latitude
- Severe sunburn during childhood

Signs and Symptoms
- Early: mole becomes asymmetric, has irregular borders, color changes, diameter increases
- Late: nodular, pruritic, bleeding, ulcerated lesions

Diagnostic Tests
- Alkaline phosphatase
- CBC
- Chest radiography
- CT
- Excisional or punch biopsy
- LDH
- Lymphatic mapping
- Monoclonal antibodies
- Sentinel node biopsy
- Ultrasound

Metastatic Sites
- Brain
- Bone
- Liver
- Lung
- Lymph nodes
- Skin
- Subcutaneous tissues

Treatment

- Surgery: curative resection or palliative. Primary treatment is wide resection with optional lymph node dissection as prophylaxis
- Radiation therapy is palliative and adjuvant for head, neck, and brain (600 cGy twice a week for a total dose of 3000 cGy)
- Biologics and immunomodulators used as adjuvants and for metastasis (ongoing clinical trials)
  - IL-2 (18–24 million IU/m^2 IV × 5 days) every 3 weeks.
  - IFN-α (10×10^6 U/m^2 SC 3 times a week) for 1 year.
  - Levamisole (450–800 mg/m^2 IV every 2 weeks) for 2–3 years
  - Monoclonal antibodies coupled with drugs, isotopes, cytokines, toxins
  - Tumor-specific melanoma vaccine, polyvalent and host tumor–specific
- Chemotherapy used as adjuvant and for metastatic disease
  - DTIC (250 mg/m^2 IV × 5 days) every 3 weeks
  - Taxol (250 mg/m^2 IV every 21 days; experimental)
  - CVD: vinblastine (1.6 mg/m^2 IV daily × 5 days) + DTIC (800 mg/m^2 IV on day 1) + cisplatin (20 mg/m^2 IV on day 2), repeated every 3 weeks
- Isolated limb perfusion used for satellite and in-transit metastases of extremities. Use melphalan (20–40 μg/ml of perfusate in a closed system)

Potential Problems
- Anorexia
- Anuria
- Changes in body image
- Diarrhea
- Edema
- Hypotension
- Infection at surgery site
- Mental status alterations
- Nausea
- Peripheral neuropathy
- Skin toxicity
- Vomiting

Potential Oncologic Emergencies
- Cardiac tamponade
- GI obstruction
- Meningeal carcinomatosis
- Spinal cord compression

Prognosis
- Using AJCC/UICC system, 5-year survival: Stage I, 90%; Stage II, 55%; Stage III, 14%; Stage IV, < 10%

Multiple Myeloma

Epidemiology

- Estimated 12,500 new cases per year
- Male-female ratio 1:1
- 10% of all hematologic cancers

Etiology/Risk Factors

- Blacks affected twice as often as whites
- Chromosomal translocations of the *myc* gene and genes that encode immunoglobulin
- Excessive production of IL-6
- Exposure to petroleum products, asbestos
- Genetic susceptibility
- Median age 62 years
- Possible viral etiology
- Radiation exposure

Signs and Symptoms

- Early: anemia, fatigue, malaise, recurrent infection, back pain
- Late: renal dysfunction, hypercalcemia, cytopenia, extramedullary plasmacytomas, pathologic fractures

Diagnostic Tests

- Bone scan
- Bone marrow aspiration
- CBC
- Coagulation panel
- Electrolyte panel
- ESR
- MRI
- Quantitative serum immunoglobulin (monoclonal bands)
- Serum β_2-microglobulin levels
- Skeletal radiography
- Urine analysis for Bence Jones proteins

Metastatic Sites

- Proximal humeri and femurs
- Skull
- Thoracic cage
- Vertebrae

Treatment

- Chemotherapy
  - Melphalan (8 mg/m^2 PO daily for 4 days) + prednisone (60 mg/m^2 PO daily for 4 days) every 4–6 weeks for 1–2 years.
  - Vincristine (0.4 mg per day IV) + doxorubicin (9 mg/m^2 IV per day for 4 days) + dexamethasone (20 mg/m^2 each morning for 4 days, beginning on days 1, 9, and 17)
  - Intermittent high-dose dexamethasone
- Radiation: At least 4500 cGy to solitary tumors
- Autogenic and allogeneic bone marrow transplant: too early to conclude effectiveness

Patient Problems

- Amyloidosis
- Anemia
- Bone pain
- Clotting disorders
- Generalized osteoporosis
- Hypercalcemia
- Pathologic fractures
- Recurrent infections
- Renal failure
- Serum hyperviscosity

Potential Oncologic Emergencies

- Hypercalcemia
- Septic shock
- Spinal cord compression

Prognosis

- Using the Durie-Salmon staging system, median survival (in months): Stage I, 61.2; Stage IB, IIA, IIB, 54.5; Stage IIIA, 30.1; Stage IIIB, 14.7

Nasopharyngeal Cancer

Epidemiology

- Endemic in Southern China, Southeast Asia, Alaska, Greenland, North Africa, and the Mediterranean basin
- Male-female ratio is 2:1 to 4:1
- Peak incidences, ages 15–25 and 40–60 years
- Approximately 9100 new cases per year
- Approximately 4100 deaths per year

Etiology/Risk Factors

- Tobacco use
- Alcohol consumption
- Epstein-Barr virus
- Consumption of salted fish
- Poor vitamin intake

Signs and Symptoms

- Aspiration symptoms
- Deep-seated ear pain
- Dysphagia
- Easy bleeding of the oral mucosa
- Erythroplakia
- Garbled, gurgling speech
- Leukoplakia
- Neck mass
- Repeated bleeding from nose or oral cavity
- Slow-healing sore
- Unilateral pain

Diagnostic Tests

- Biopsy
- Bone scan
- CBC
- CT
- Chest radiography
- Complete head and neck exam
- Dental consult
- Panendoscopy
- Serum chemistries
- Videoendoscopic exam

Metastatic Sites

- Bone
- Brain
- Liver
- Lung
- Regional lymph nodes

Treatment

- Radiation therapy is the treatment of choice; early-stage lesions receive 6600 cGy and advanced lesions 7000 cGy

Potential Problems

- Altered sense of smell
- Anorexia
- Anxiety
- Body image disturbance
- Decreased nutritional intake
- Dental problems
- Dysphagia
- Grieving
- Impaired verbal communication
- Ineffective breathing pattern
- Pain
- Stomatitis
- Taste changes
- Xerostomia

Potential Oncologic Emergencies

- Airway obstruction
- Pneumonia

Prognosis

- 5- and 10-year survival rates 36–62%

Neuroblastoma

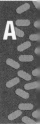

Epidemiology
- Most common extracranial solid tumor of childhood
- Accounts for 8–10% of all pediatric cancers
- 550 new cases per year
- Median age at diagnosis is 2 years

Etiology/Risk Factors
- Familial history
- Neurofibromatosis
- Hirschsprung's disease
- Beckwith-Wiedemann syndrome
- Fetal hydantoin syndrome

Signs and Symptoms
- Abdominal mass
- Bone pain
- Failure to gain weight
- Fever
- Hard, painless mass in the neck
- Horner's syndrome
- Malaise
- Pain
- Periorbital ecchymoses
- Scalp nodules
- Thoracic mass

Diagnostic Tests
- Abdominal ultrasound
- Bone scan
- Bone marrow biopsy
- BUN and creatinine
- CT
- Chest radiography
- Coagulation profile
- CBC
- Liver enzymes
- MRI
- Serum ferritin level
- Serum GD_2-ganglioside level
- Serum NSE levels
- Skeletal radiography
- Urinanalysis
- Urinary catecholamines

Metastatic Sites
- Bone
- Bone marrow
- Liver
- Lung
- Lymph nodes
- Orbit
- Skin

Treatment
- Surgery used in patients with tumors localized to one side of the midline without encasement of major blood vessels
- Radiation therapy useful for localized but unresectable tumors
- Chemotherapy is the primary treatment involving combination regimens (e.g., cyclophosphamide and doxorubicin; cisplatin and etoposide)

Potential Problems
- Anxiety
- Diarrhea
- Fatigue
- Fever
- Impaired mobility
- Ineffective family coping
- Infection
- Nausea and vomiting
- Nutritional deficit
- Pain

Potential Oncologic Emergencies
- Intestinal obstruction
- Pathologic fractures
- Septic shock
- Spinal cord compression

Prognosis
- Overall survival: Stage I, 90%; Stage 2A, 80%; Stage 2B or 3, 60%

Non-Hodgkin's Lymphoma

Epidemiology
- Approximately 40,000 cases per year in the United States
- Increased incidence in elders

Etiology/Risk Factors
- Altered immune status: AIDS, organ transplantation, rheumatoid arthritis, inherited immune deficiencies
- Virus: HTLV, HIV, Epstein-Barr
- Chemical exposure
- Radiation exposure

Signs and Symptoms
- Abdominal mass
- Adenopathy
- Fatigue
- Malaise
- Night sweats
- Splenomegaly
- Unexplained fever
- Weight loss

Diagnostic Tests
- Bone marrow biopsy
- Bone scan
- CBC
- CT
- Liver biopsy
- Liver enzymes
- Lymph node biopsy
- MRI
- Serum albumin level
- Serum bilirubin
- Serum LDH level
- Splenic biopsy
- Uric acid level

Metastatic Sites
- Bone
- Liver
- Lung

Treatment

- Low-grade (i.e., less aggressive) lymphoma: patients generally have widespread disease at the time of diagnosis. Many clinicians adapt an approach of watchful waiting with these patients, whereas others recommend combination chemotherapy regimens (e.g., CVP [cyclophosphamide, vincristine, prednisone], COPP [cyclophosphamide, vincristine, procarbazine, prednisone], or CHOP [cyclophosphamide, doxorubicin, vincristine, prednisone])
- Intermediate/high-grade lymphoma treated with combination chemotherapy, with or without radiation therapy. Current combination regimens include these:
  - BACOP: bleomycin (5 U/m^2 IV on days 15 and 22), doxorubicin (25 mg/m^2 IV on days 1 and 8), cyclophosphamide (650 mg/m^2 IV on days 1 and 8), vincristine (1.4 mg/m^2 IV on days 1 and 8 [not to exceed 2.0 mg]), and prednisone (60 mg/m^2 PO on days 15–28) repeat every 28 days
  - COMLA: cyclophosphamide (1500 mg/m^2 IV on day 1), vincristine (1.4 mg/m^2 IV on days 1, 8, 15 [not to exceed 25 mg]), methotrexate (120 mg/m^2 IV on days 22, 29, 36, 43, 50, 57, 64, 71), leucovorin (25 mg/m^2 PO q6hr, for four doses starting 24 hours after each methotrexate dose), and cytarabine (300 mg/m^2 IV on days 22, 29, 36, 43, 50, 57, 64, 71); repeat every 91 days

Potential Problems
- Depression
- Fatigue
- Fever
- Infection
- Mucositis
- Nausea and vomiting
- Nutritional deficit
- Pain

Potential Oncologic Emergencies
- Septic shock
- Spinal cord compression
- Tumor lysis syndrome

Prognosis
- Low-grade lymphoma is rarely curable; however, survival ranges from 4–8 years, with or without treatment
- Intermediate/high-grade lymphomas: localized disease is curable in 75% of patients; disseminated disease is curable in 30–40% of patients

Oropharyngeal Cancer

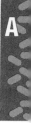

Epidemiology
- Approximately 28,150 new cases per year
- Approximately 8370 deaths per year

Etiology/Risk Factors
- Tobacco use
- Alcohol consumption
- Pipe and cigar smokers
- Chewing tobacco
- Oral snuff
- Vitamin A deficiency
- Poor oral hygiene
- Chronic periodontitis
- Viral superinfection
- Ill-fitting dentures

Signs and Symptoms
- Aspiration symptoms
- Deep-seated ear pain
- Dysphagia
- Easy bleeding of the mucosal surface
- Erythroplakia
- Leukoplakia
- Neck mass
- Repeated bleeding from the mouth
- Slow-healing sore
- Trismus
- Unilateral pain

Diagnostic Tests
- Biopsy
- Bone scan
- CBC
- CT
- Chest radiography
- Complete head and neck exam
- Dental consult
- Panendoscopy
- Serum chemistries
- Videoendoscopy

Metastatic Sites
- Bone
- Brain
- Liver
- Lung
- Regional lymph nodes

Treatment

- Primary treatment for early-stage disease (T1; T2N0) is radiation therapy or surgery. Because of the extensive lymphatic network in the oropharynx, 75% of patients present with lymph node involvement
- Surgery may involve total laryngectomy
- With more advanced disease (T3, T4) the management plan typically involves radiation therapy alone or surgery followed by radiation therapy

Potential Problems
- Altered sense of smell
- Anorexia
- Anxiety
- Body image disturbance
- Decreased nutritional intake
- Dental problems
- Dysphagia
- Grieving
- Impaired verbal communication
- Ineffective breathing pattern
- Pain
- Stomatitis
- Taste changes
- Xerostomia

Potential Oncologic Emergencies
- Airway obstruction
- Carotid hemorrhage
- Pneumonia

Prognosis
- Prognosis varies depending on the anatomic location of the tumor and the stage of the disease; overall cure rate < 50%

Osteogenic Sarcoma

Epidemiology
- 2070 new cases per year
- 0.2% of all new cancers
- Male-female ratio 1.1:1

Etiology/Risk Factors
- Age 13.5 for girls and 14.5 for boys
- Rapid bone growth
- Hereditary retinoblastoma
- History of another primary malignancy
- History of trauma
- Paget's disease
- Prior irradiation of the bone
- Taller stature

Signs and Symptoms
- Early: pain, palpable mass, swelling, limited motion
- Late: fractures, anorexia, weight loss

Diagnostic Tests
- Arteriography
- Biopsy and histologic examination
- CT or MRI
- Radiography

Metastatic Sites
- Adrenals
- Brain
- Bone
- Kidney
- Lung
- Pericardium
- Pleura

Treatment

- Surgery: removal of all gross and microscopic tumor; amputation versus limb-sparing
- Radiation therapy used for pain control and to prevent and control pulmonary metastases
- Adjuvant chemotherapy
  - High-dose methotrexate (12 g/m^2 IV with leucovorin rescue $\times$ 1) on weeks 4, 5, 6, 7, 11, 12, 15, 16, 29, 30, 44, 45
  - Cyclophosphamide (600 mg/m^2 IV) + bleomycin (15 mg/m^2 IV) + actinomycin D (0.6 mg/m^2 $\times$ 2) on weeks 2, 13, 26, 39, 42
  - Doxorubicin (30 mg/m^2 IV $\times$ 3)
  - Doxorubicin (50 mg/m^2 IV) + cisplatin (100 mg/m^2 IV $\times$ 1) on weeks 20, 22, 33, 36

Potential Problems
- Amputation
- Anorexia
- Changes in body image
- Dehydration
- Electrolyte imbalance
- Infection
- Stomatitis
- Weight loss

Potential Oncological Emergencies
- Hypercalcemia

Prognosis
- Disease-free survival of 5 years 54–76%, depending on the treatment

Ovarian Cancer: Epithelial

Epidemiology

- 24,000 new cases per year
- 4% of all female cancers

Etiology/Risk Factors

- Age range 40–70; peaks at 70 years
- Asbestos exposure
- High-fat diet
- Infertility
- Late child bearing
- Nulliparity
- History of breast cancer
- Family history
- Whites > blacks
- Urban dwelling

Signs and Symptoms

- Early: frequently asymptomatic or vague abdominal symptoms (mild indigestion, urinary abnormalities, abdominal discomfort)
- Late: hemorrhage (from necrotic tumor), sepsis, profound cachexia, gastrointestinal obstruction, ascites

Diagnostic Tests

- BUN and creatinine
- CA-125
- CBC
- CT
- Exploratory laparotomy
- MRI
- Paracentesis
- Vaginal ultrasound

Metastatic Sites

- Bladder
- Bone
- CNS
- Lung
- Lymph nodes (paraaortic, supraclavicular, axillary, inguinal, diaphragmatic)
- Peritoneum
- Sigmoid colon
- Small intestine
- Uterus

Treatment

- Surgery
  - Total abdominal hysterectomy and bilateral salpingo-oophorectomy as curative resection
  - Second-look laparotomy as a curative or evaluative procedure
- Chemotherapy
  - Melphalan (0.2 mg/kg per day) for 5 of every 28 days
  - CAP: cyclophosphamide (300 mg/m^2 IV on day 1) + doxorubicin (30 mg/m^2 IV on day 1) + cisplatin (50 mg/m^2 IV on day 1)
  - MAC: mitomycin (7 mg/m^2 IV) + doxorubicin (45 mg/m^2 IV) + cyclophosphamide (450 mg/m^2 IV)
  - Carboplatin (350 to 400 mg/m^2)
  - Paclitaxel (135 mg/m^2 as a 24-hour infusion every 3 weeks) + cisplatin (75 mg/m^2) administered after paclitaxel
- Radiation used as adjuvant therapy
  - Whole-abdomen and pelvic radiation: open-field technique of entire peritoneal cavity, 2000–3000 cGy in fractions of 100–125 cGy, the pelvis is boosted in 180-cGy fractions to a total of 5000 cGy
  - Intraperitoneal radiocolloid phosphorus 32.
- Biologics currently investigational

Potential Problems

- Anxiety
- Chemotherapy-related toxicities
- Fertility issues
- Fluid and electrolyte imbalance
- Nausea and vomiting
- Nutrition
- Pain
- Sexual dysfunction

Potential Oncologic Emergencies

- DIC
- Ureteral obstruction

Prognosis

- Using AJCC/UICC system, 5-year survival: Stage I, ≤ 90%; Stage II, ≤ 70%; Stage III, 25%; Stage IV, 10%

Ovarian Cancer: Stromal and Germ Cell

Epidemiology
- 5% of all ovarian cancers

Etiology/Risk Factors
- Age range 40–70; peaks at 70 years
- Asbestos exposure
- High-fat diet
- Infertility
- Late child bearing
- Nulliparity
- History of breast cancer
- Positive family history
- Whites > blacks
- Urbanization

Signs and Symptoms
- Early: frequently asymptomatic or vague abdominal symptoms (mild indigestion, urinary abnormalities, abdominal discomfort)
- Late: hemorrhage (from necrotized tumor), sepsis, profound cachexia, gastrointestinal obstruction, ascites

Diagnostic Tests
- α-Fetoprotein level
- BUN and creatinine
- CA-125
- CBC
- CT
- Exploratory laparotomy
- HCG level
- MRI
- Paracentesis
- Vaginal ultrasound

Metastatic Sites
- Bladder
- Bone
- CNS
- Lung
- Lymph nodes (paraaortic, supraclavicular, axillary, inguinal, diaphragmatic)
- Peritoneum
- Sigmoid colon
- Small intestine
- Uterus

Treatment
- Stages I to III: complete resection of disease; adjuvant chemotherapy (either bleomycin, etoposide, and cisplatin *or* vincristine, actinomycin, and cyclophosphamide)
- Stage III to IV disease that is incompletely resected; systemic therapy with bleomycin, etoposide, and cisplatin with close follow-up evaluations

Potential Problems
- Anxiety
- Chemotherapy-related toxicities
- Fertility issues
- Fluid and electrolyte imbalance
- Nausea and vomiting
- Nutrition
- Pain
- Sexual dysfunction

Potential Oncologic Emergencies
- DIC
- Ureteral obstruction

Prognosis
- Prognosis is variable, depending on the stage of the disease at the time of diagnosis

Pancreatic Cancer

Epidemiology
- 27,000 new cases per year
- More common in males

Etiology/Risk Factors
- Age > 50
- Chronic pancreatitis
- Cigarette smoking
- Diabetes mellitus
- Excessive intake of coffee, alcohol, dietary fat
- Exposure to dry-cleaning chemicals, coke, industrial pollutants
- Lower economic status
- Black-white ratio 1.5:1

Signs and Symptoms
- Early: insidious and nonspecific or none
- Late: pain, weight loss, altered bowel habits, diarrhea, greasy stools, severe constipation, jaundice, sudden onset of diabetes

Diagnostic Tests
- Abdominal ultrasound
- Alkaline phosphatase
- Bilirubin
- CA 19-9
- CBC
- CT
- Chest radiography
- ERCP
- Hepatic transaminases
- Laparotomy
- MRI
- PTC
- Serum CEA
- Serum lipase

Metastatic Sites
- Adjacent large vessels
- Bile duct
- Duodenum
- Lymph nodes
- Spleen
- Stomach
- Transverse colon

Treatment

- Surgery
  - Pancreaticoduodenectomy (Whipple procedure) as curative or palliative resection
  - Regional (total) pancreatectomy as curative resection
  - Distal pancreatectomy as curative resection
  - Surgical bypass procedures: transhepatic percutaneous biliary bypass and endoscopic stent placement as palliative procedures
- Chemotherapy
  - FAM: 5-FU (600 mg/m^2 per week IV on weeks 1, 2, 5, 6, 9) + doxorubicin (30 mg/m^2 per week IV on weeks 1, 5, 9) + mitomycin (10 mg/m^2 per week on weeks 1, 9); repeat every 8 weeks
  - SMF: streptozotocin (1000 mg/m^2 IV on days 1, 8, 29, 36) + 5-FU (600 mg/m^2 IV on days 1, 8, 29, 36) + mitomycin (10 mg/m^2 IV on day 1); repeat every 8 weeks
- Adjuvant radiation therapy:
  - External radiation used to reduce symptoms (4000 cGy over 6 weeks)
  - Intraoperative radiation therapy (2000 cGy immediately after resection)
  - External beam radiation therapy for palliation of pain (three-field approach and fractions of 180–200 cGy)
- Biologics under clinical investigation

Potential Problems
- Malabsorption
- Malnutrition
- Pain

Potential Oncologic Emergencies
- Biliary tract obstruction
- Gastric outlet obstruction
- Small bowel obstruction

Prognosis
- 3-year survival rate: Stage I, 15% in patients with resected tumors of the pancreas and 1% in all other patients; Stage II, 2%; Stage III, < 2%; Stage IV, < 1%

Prostate Cancer

Epidemiology
- 244,000 new cases per year
- Accounts for 36% of new cancers in men

Etiology/Risk Factors
- Age > 50 years (incidence increases with age)
- Factors related to endogenous hormones (testosterone)
- High-fat diet
- History of vasectomy
- Family history of prostate and/or breast cancer
- Race (black > white > Asian)

Signs and Symptoms
- Early: urinary urgency, frequency, hesitancy, nocturia, new onset of impotence or less firm penile erections
- Late: bone pain (most commonly due to vertebral metastases)

Diagnostic Tests
- Abdominal pelvic CT
- Biopsy (core needle, fine-needle aspiration, open, or transurethral)
- CBC, BUN, creatinine, liver function
- Digital rectal exam
- Pelvic lymphadenectomy (open or laparoscopic)
- Radionuclide bone scan
- Serum PSA
- Transrectal ultrasonography
- Urinalysis

Metastatic Sites
- Bone (most common site of distant metastases)
- Liver
- Lungs

Treatment
- Close observation (watchful waiting): for men with low-grade, low-stage disease with a life expectancy < 10 years
- Surgery
  - Radical prostatectomy: for localized disease (Stage A or B); nerve-sparing technique, which preserves erectile function in many men, may be used for early-stage tumors
  - Transurethral resection of the prostate (TURP): for bladder outlet obstruction when radical prostatectomy is not an option; no curative potential
- Radiation therapy for localized disease (Stage A or B) and when tumor is localized to periprostatic area (Stage C); external-beam therapy is used more frequently than interstitial radiation, owing to superior results; external-beam also used for palliative treatment of soft tissue and osseous metastases
- Hormone therapy used primarily for metastatic disease (Stage D) with orchiectomy; option for earlier-stage disease when more aggressive therapy is contraindicated
  - Diethylstilbestrol (3–5 mg/day)
  - Leuprolide (1.0 mg/day SC)
  - Leuprolide depot (7.5 mg IM monthly)
  - Goserelin depot (3.6 mg SC monthly)
  - Leuprolide (1.0 mg/day SC) + flutamide (250 mg, t.i.d.)
- Chemotherapy for hormonally refractory disease
  - Adriamycin (60 mg/m^2 IV every 3 weeks)
  - Cyclophosphamide (1 g/m^2 IV every 3 weeks)
  - 5-FU (500 mg/m^2 IV weekly)
  - Methotrexate (40 mg/m^2 IV weekly)
  - Cisplatin (40 mg/m^2 IV every 3 weeks)

Potential Problems
- Bone marrow suppression
- Cardiovascular complications
- Cystitis
- Decreased libido
- Diarrhea
- Enteritis
- Gynecomastia
- Hematuria
- Hot flashes
- Impotence
- Incontinence
- Proctitis
- Rectal anal stricture
- Rectal bleeding
- Rectal ulcer
- Scrotal or lower extremity edema
- Urethral stricture
- Urinary retention

Potential Oncologic Emergencies
- Bowel obstruction
- DIC
- Meningeal carcinomatosis
- Spinal cord compression
- SIADH

Prognosis
- Using Jewett staging system, 5-year progression-free survival with treatment: Stage A1, equivalent to general population for men > 70 years; Stage A2, > 90%; Stage B1, 85%

Rectal Cancer

Epidemiology

- Second most common malignant tumor
- Approximately 60,000 new cases per year
- Approximately 61,000 deaths
- 62% of the lesions occur distally

Etiology/Risk Factors

- Familial polyposis
- Chronic ulcerative colitis
- Family cancer syndrome
- Increasing age

Signs and Symptoms

- Abdominal pain
- Change in bowel habit
- Jaundice
- Malaise
- Obstipation
- Obstruction
- Occult blood
- Pelvic pain
- Rectal bleeding
- Tenesmus

Diagnostic Tests

- Barium enema
- CEA level
- Chest radiography
- Colonoscopy
- Cytoscopy
- Digital rectal examination
- Fecal occult blood test
- Intravenous pyelogram
- Liver scan
- Rectal ultrasound
- Sigmoidoscopy

Metastatic Sites

- Liver
- Lungs
- Lymph nodes

Treatment

- Surgery: procedures vary, depending on the location and size of the tumor and range from local excision to abdominal perineal resection
- Preoperative radiation therapy (30–60 cGy) may be of some benefit

Potential Problems

- Altered bowel elimination
- Body image disturbance
- Impaired sexual functioning
- Infection
- Nutritional deficit
- Pain

Potential Oncologic Emergencies

- Intestinal obstruction
- Septic shock

Prognosis

- 5-year survival rate approximately 50%

Salivary Gland Tumors

Epidemiology
• Higher incidence in Eskimos

Etiology/Risk Factors
• Radiation exposure

Signs and Symptoms
• Deep-seated ear pain
• Easy bleeding of the mucosal surface
• Erythroplakia
• Leukoplakia
• Neck mass
• Slow-healing sore

Diagnostic Tests
• Biopsy
• Bone scan
• CBC
• CT
• Chest radiography
• Complete head and neck examination
• Dental consult
• Panendoscopy
• Serum chemistries
• Videoendoscopic exam

Metastatic Sites
• Bone
• Brain
• Liver
• Lung
• Regional lymph nodes

Treatment

• Treatment usually involves surgical excision followed by postoperative radiation therapy

Potential Problems
• Altered sense of smell
• Anorexia
• Anxiety
• Body image disturbance
• Decreased nutritional intake
• Dental problems
• Dysphagia
• Grieving
• Impaired verbal communication
• Ineffective breathing pattern
• Pain
• Stomatitis
• Taste changes
• Xerostomia

Potential Oncologic Emergencies
• Airway obstruction
• Pneumonia

Prognosis
• Patients can live 10–20 years following diagnosis

Sarcoma: Soft Tissue

Epidemiology

- 5800 new cases per year
- Incidence 2 in 100,000 persons
- Approximately 0.7% of all cancers
- Fifth most common cancer in children < 15 years

Etiology/Risk Factors

- Family history of breast cancer
- Foreign body implantations
- Genetic predisposition
- History of exposure to radiation
- Recent history of trauma

Signs and Symptoms

- Early: asymptomatic soft tissue mass
- Late: symptoms result from pressure or traction on adjacent nerves or muscles

Diagnostic Tests

- Biopsy (incisional or excisional)
- Bone scan
- CT of affected region
- CT of lung
- MRI
- Soft tissue radiograph
- Ultrasound

Metastatic Sites

- Lung
- Lymph nodes

Treatment

- Surgery usually the primary treatment, with or without radiation therapy with wide excision
- Radiation therapy may be administered preoperatively or postoperatively
- Chemotherapy may be used as adjuvant therapy and is used with metastatic disease
  - CyADIC regimen: cyclophosphamide (600 mg/m^2 IV on day 1) + doxorubicin (15 mg/m^2/24 hours for 4 days as continuous IV infusion) + dacarbazine (250 mg/m^2/24 hours for 4 days as continuous IV infusion); repeat cycle every 3–4 weeks
  - ADIC regimen: doxorubicin (22.5 mg/m^2/24 hours for 4 days as continuous IV infusion) + dacarbazine (225 mg/m^2/24 hours for 4 days as continuous IV infusion); repeat cycle every 3–4 weeks
  - MAID regimen: Mesna (10,000 mg/m^2/24 hours for 4 days as continuous IV infusion) + doxorubicin (20 mg/m^2/24 hours for 3 days as continuous IV infusion) + ifosfamide (2500 mg/m^2/24 hours for 3 days as continuous IV infusion) + dacarbazine (250 mg/m^2/24 hours for 4 days as continuous IV infusion), repeat every 3 to 4 weeks

Potential Problems

- Alopecia
- Body image changes
- Cardiac toxicity
- Fever
- Hemorrhagic cystitis
- Infection
- Mucositis
- Nausea and vomiting
- Neutropenia
- Thrombocytopenia

Potential Oncologic Emergencies

- Pleural effusions
- Sepsis

Prognosis

- 5-year survival: Stage I, 75%; Stage 2, 55%; Stage III, 29%; Stage IV, < 10%

Skin Cancer: Basal Cell

Epidemiology
- Most common cancer among whites
- 600,000 new cases per year
- Men > women

Etiology/Risk Factors
- Advanced age
- Basal cell nevus syndrome
- Excessive sun exposure
- Fair skin, blue eyes, fair hair
- Radiation exposure
- Temperate climate
- Traumatic injury
- Xeroderma pigmentosa

Signs and Symptoms
- Early: slow-growing, shiny, skin-colored to pink, translucent, raised papule with telangiectasia
- Late: ulcerated lesion with rolled border and crusted center

Diagnostic Tests
- Biopsy
- Skin examination

Metastatic Sites
- Local invasion into skin, cartilage, soft tissue, and bone
- Rarely metastasizes

Treatment

- Surgery
  - For smaller lesions, surgical excision or curettage and dissection
  - For tumors with ill-defined margins and for recurrent tumors, Moh's micrographic surgery
- Radiation therapy used for basal cell carcinoma of the eyelid, nose, and lips
- Chemotherapy (5-FU cream [5%])
- Biologics: serial intralesional injections of IFN

Potential Problems
- Body image change
- Knowledge deficit

Potential Oncologic Emergencies
- None

Prognosis
- Excellent when person avoids excessive sun exposure

Skin Cancer: Squamous Cell Carcinoma

Epidemiology

- Men > women
- Incidence 166 in 100,000 persons

Etiology/Risk Factors

- Albinism
- Chronic sinus disease
- Chronic ulceration
- Excessive sun exposure
- Exposure to cotton oil, arsenic
- Exposure to human papillomavirus
- Fair skin
- Immunosuppressive therapy
- Radiation exposure
- Trauma/burns
- Treatment with PUVA

Signs and Symptoms

- Early: red, indurated papule that appears de novo or on an actinic keratosis and expands rapidly, producing a large nodule
- Late: ulceration and metastasis of lesion to lymph node

Diagnostic Tests

- Biopsy
- Skin examination

Metastatic Sites

- Lymph nodes

Treatment

- Surgery: wide excision, with or without Moh's procedure
- Chemotherapy: topical 5% fluorouracil for superficial squamous cell carcinoma

Potential Problems

- Body image change
- Knowledge deficit

Potential Oncologic Emergencies

- None

Prognosis

- The higher the number of undifferentiated cells, the worse is the prognosis; however, prognosis is excellent when the patient avoids excessive sun exposure

Small Intestine Cancer: Adenocarcinoma

Epidemiology
- 45% of all malignant small bowel cancers
- Distributed in duodenum or jejunum
- Males > females

Etiology/Risk Factors
- Age 70+ years
- Celiac disease
- Crohn's disease
- Familial adenomatous polyposis
- High-fat intake
- Peutz-Jeghers syndrome
- von Recklinghausen's neurofibromatosis

Signs and Symptoms
- Early: pain, weight loss
- Late: bleeding, perforation, palpable mass, anemia, hyperbilirubinemia

Diagnostic Tests
- Abdominal radiography
- Barium enema
- CBC
- CT
- Endoscopy
- Liver function tests
- Serum bilirubin
- Upper GI series

Metastatic Sites
- Liver
- Lymph nodes

Treatment
- Surgery: pancreaticoduodenectomy for tumors of the first or second portion of duodenum; segmental duodenectomy and anastomosis for tumors of the third or fourth portion of the duodenum
- Radiation therapy for palliation
- Chemotherapy: investigational protocols with 5-FU

Potential Problems
- Altered body image
- Anemia
- Anorexia
- Diarrhea
- Fatigue
- Fluid and electrolyte imbalance
- Pain
- Pruritus
- Weight loss

Potential Oncologic Emergencies
- Intestinal obstruction
- Sepsis

Prognosis
- Survival rates poor: only 20–30% of patients are alive after 5 years

Small Intestine Cancer: Lymphoma

Epidemiology

- 17% of all small bowel malignancies
- May be a manifestation of disseminated systemic disease
- Incidence increases with distal progression
- Ileum is most frequent site

Etiology/Risk Factors

- Age 54–61 years
- Crohn's disease
- High-fat intake
- Males > females

Signs and Symptoms

- Early: abdominal pain associated with partial bowel obstruction, abdominal mass
- Late: anemia, perforation

Diagnostic Tests

- Abdominal radiography
- Barium enema
- CBC
- Colonoscopy
- CT
- Endoscopy
- Laparotomy
- Upper GI series

Metastatic Sites

- Bone marrow
- Lymph nodes
- Spleen

Treatment

- Surgery: bowel resection with removal of the mesentery
- Radiation therapy may be used

Potential Problems

- Anemia
- Anorexia
- Diarrhea
- Fatigue
- Pain
- Weight loss

Potential Oncologic Emergencies

- Intestinal obstruction
- Sepsis

Prognosis

- 5-year survival 10–76%

Small Intestine Cancer: Sarcoma

Epidemiology

- 11% of all small bowel cancers
- Most are of smooth muscle origin
- Males > females

Etiology/Risk Factors

- Age 70+ years
- Celiac disease
- Crohn's disease
- Familial adenomatous polyps
- High-fat intake
- Peutz-Jeghers syndrome
- von Recklinghausen's neurofibromatosis

Signs and Symptoms

- Early: bleeding, obstruction, abdominal mass
- Late: perforation, anemia

Diagnostic Tests

- Abdominal radiography
- CBC
- CT
- Endoscopy
- Liver function tests
- Serum bilirubin
- Upper GI series

Metastatic Sites

- Liver
- Peritoneum

Treatment

- Surgery: wedge resection for smaller lesions, pancreaticoduodenectomy, or segmental resection (including the supporting mesentery)
- Chemotherapy to treat symptomatic metastatic disease

Potential Problems

- Altered body image
- Anemia
- Anorexia
- Diarrhea
- Fatigue
- Fluid and electrolyte imbalance
- Pain
- Pruritus
- Weight loss

Potential Oncologic Emergencies

- Intestinal obstruction
- Sepsis

Prognosis

- 5-year survival 10–50%

Stomach Cancer

Epidemiology

- Ninth among causes of death among males and fifteenth among females in the United States
- Male-female ratio 2.2:1
- High incidence in Japan, China, Iceland, and portions of Central and South America

Etiology/Risk Factors

- Adenomatous polyps
- Blood group A carries more risk than group O
- Colder climates
- Diet: pickled uncooked vegetables, salty sauces, and dried, salted fish
- Lower socioeconomic class
- Pernicious anemia
- Family history
- History of ulcer surgery
- Smoking
- Occupational exposure to nickel, rubber, and asbestos

Signs and Symptoms

- Early: a vague, uneasy sense of fullness, a feeling of heaviness, moderate distention after meals
- Late: weight loss, loss of appetite, nausea and vomiting, weakness, fatigue, anemia

Diagnostic Tests

- Barium enema
- CBC
- Endoscopy with biopsies
- Fecal occult blood
- Tumor markers (CA50, CEA, TPA)
- Upper GI series

Metastatic Sites

- Bone
- Duodenum
- Esophagus
- Intraperitoneum
- Liver
- Lung
- Pancreas
- Regional lymph nodes

Treatment

- Surgery: subtotal gastrectomy or total gastrectomy (even more radical approach, with extended lymph node dissection and extended regional resection of the liver, spleen, pancreas, or transverse colon)
- Radiation therapy used in combination with surgery and chemotherapy, preoperatively, intraoperatively, or postoperatively (usual dose 4000–5000 cGy over 4 to 5 weeks)
- Chemotherapy: 5-FU, mitomycin C, carmustine, methyl-CCNU, doxorubicin, cisplatin
- Combination chemotherapy:
  - 5-FU (600 mg/m^2 IV on days 1, 8, 29, and 36) + doxorubicin (30 mg/m^2 IV on days 1 and 29) + mitomycin (10 mg/m^2 IV on day 1)
    or
  - Doxorubicin (20 mg/m^2 IV on days 1 and 7) + cisplatin (40 mg/m^2 on days 2 and 8) + etoposide (120 mg/m^2 IV on days 4, 5, and 6); repeat cycle every 3–4 weeks
    or
  - Doxorubicin (20 mg/m^2 IV on days 1 and 8) + cisplatin (40 mg/m^2 IV on days 2 and 8) + etoposide (100 mg/m^2 IV on days 1–3); repeat cycle every 4 weeks

Potential Problems

- Anastomotic leak
- Anxiety
- Dehydration
- Diarrhea/constipation
- Dumping syndrome
- Fatigue
- Malnutrition
- Nausea/vomiting
- Steatorrhea
- Vitamin B$_{12}$ deficiency
- Weight loss

Potential Oncologic Emergencies

- Gastric outlet obstruction
- Intestinal obstruction

Prognosis

- 5-year survival rate: Stage I, 85%; Stage II with regional lymph nodes involvement, 25%
- Disseminated disease: weeks to months

Testicular Cancer: Not Seminoma

Epidemiology
- Contains embryonal, teratocarcinoma, teratoma, and choriocarcinoma cells

Etiology
- Carcinogenesis probably begins in utero through exposure to maternal estrogen
- Process is reactivated at puberty by endogenous male hormones

Risk Factors
- Age: peaks in infants, young adults (20–40 years), and older adults (> 60 years)
- Excess maternal weight during pregnancy
- Exogenous hormone replacement during mother's pregnancy
- Offspring of first pregnancy
- Undescended testicles
- White race

Signs and Symptoms
- Early: painless swelling or nodule in one testis; dull ache
- Late: evidence of metastatic disease, back pain, neck pain, respiratory symptoms, GI symptoms

Diagnostic Tests
- Abdominal CT
- AFP level
- Chest radiography
- HCG levels
- Histologic examination of testis after orchiectomy
- LDH
- Testicular examination
- Transillumination (tumor does not transilluminate)
- Ultrasound

Metastatic Sites
- CNS
- Lymph nodes
- Lung

Treatment
- Surgery: orchiectomy and RPLND for Stage I and minimal Stage II disease; orchiectomy, with or without RPNLD, for advanced Stage II and Stage III disease
- Follow-up: patients should be followed with chest radiography, α-fetoprotein level and β-HCG level monthly for the first year and every other month for the second year
- Chemotherapy for advanced Stage II and Stage III disease
  - Bleomycin + etoposide + cisplatin
  - Vinblastine + ifosfamide + cisplatin
- Autologous bone marrow transplantation may be used for progressive disease

Potential Problems
- Anorexia
- Changes in body image
- Infection
- Infertility
- Sterility
- Stomatitis

Potential Oncologic Emergencies
- Pleural effusion
- Spinal cord compression

Prognosis
- 5-year survival: Stage I, > 95%; Stage II, > 95%; Stage III, > 70%

Testicular Cancer: Seminomas

Epidemiology

- 7100 new cases per year in United States
- 1.05% of male cancers
- 0.57% of all cancers

Etiology

- Carcinogenesis probably begins in utero through exposure to maternal estrogen
- Process is reactivated at puberty by endogenous male hormones

Risk Factors

- Age: peaks in infants; young adults (20–40 years); and older adults (> 60 years)
- Excess maternal weight during pregnancy
- Exogenous hormone treatment during pregnancy
- Offspring of first pregnancy
- Undescended testis
- White race

Signs and Symptoms

- Early: painless swelling or nodule in one testis; dull ache
- Late: evidence of metastatic disease, back pain, neck pain, respiratory symptoms, GI symptoms

Diagnostic Tests

- Abdominal CT
- AFP level
- Chest radiography
- HCG level
- Histologic exam of testis after orchiectomy
- LDH level
- Testicular exam
- Transillumination (tumor does not transilluminate)
- Ultrasound

Metastatic Sites

- CNS
- Lymph nodes
- Lungs

Treatment

- Surgery: orchiectomy for Stage I, II, or III
- Adjuvant radiation therapy following orchiectomy in Stage I and II disease
- Chemotherapy for bulky Stage II or III disease
  - VAB-VI: vinblastine (4 mg/m^2) + cyclophosphamide (600 mg/m^2) + dactinomycin (1 mg/m^2) + bleomycin (30 U IV on day 1, then 20 U/m^2 continuous IV infusion on days 1–3) + cisplatin (120 mg/m^2 on day 4), administered every 4 weeks for three courses
  - PVB: cisplatin (20 mg/m^2 × 5 days every 3 weeks × 4) + vinblastine (0.15 mg/kg on days 1 and 2, every 3 weeks × 4) + bleomycin (30 U weekly × 12)
  - PVP-16B: cisplatin (20 mg/m^2 × 5 days every 3 weeks × 4) + VP-16 (100 mg/m^2 × 5 days every 3 weeks × 4) + bleomycin (30 U weekly × 12)
  - For bulky Stage II or III disease with metastases (retroperitoneal nodes, lung, liver, bone, brain): cisplatin (20 mg/m^2 IV on days 1 and 5) + etoposide (75 mg/m^2 IV on days 1 and 5) + ifosfamide (1200 mg/m^2 IV on days 1 through 5 with mesna); repeat every 3 weeks
- BMT: experimental treatment for refractory disease

Potential Problems

- Anorexia
- Changes in body image
- Infection
- Infertility
- Sterility
- Stomatitis

Potential Oncologic Emergencies

- Pleural effusion
- Spinal cord compression

Prognosis

- 5-year survival: Stage I, > 95%; Stage II, > 95%; Stage III, 70%

Thyroid Cancer

Epidemiology

- 13,000 new cases per year
- 1% of all cancers
- Male-female ratio 1:3

Etiology/Risk Factors

- Age < 20 or > 60
- Autoimmune thyroiditis
- Chronic elevation of TSH
- Familial syndromes: MEN syndrome, Cowden's disease, Gardner's syndrome
- Family history of thyroid cancer
- Iodine abuse or deficiency
- Pregnancy
- Radiation exposure to head and neck during childhood

Signs and Symptoms

- Early: small, solitary nodule in thyroid gland
- Late: hoarseness, dysphagia, respiratory distress, cervical lymphadenopathies

Diagnostic Tests

- Barium swallow
- Core needle biopsy
- Fine-needle aspiration
- MRI
- Radioactive iodine/technetium scan
- TSH, T_4, T_3, calcitonin levels
- Ultrasound

Metastatic Sites

- Bone
- Brain
- Liver
- Lung

Treatment

- Surgery: total or subtotal thyroidectomy, as primary treatment, may be curative or palliative
- Radiation therapy used for ablation of postsurgical remnants and metastatic disease
  - I^{131} (101 mCi, PO) every 6–12 months for a total dose of 500 mCi
  - External beam for palliation of tumor (total dose 5600 cGy)
- Hormonal: used to control a TSH-driven tumor
  - TSH suppression therapy with L-thyroxine
- Chemotherapy used for advanced, refractory thyroid cancer
  - Doxorubicin (45–75 mg/m^2 IV); repeat every 3 weeks
  - Doxorubicin (60 mg/m^2 IV) + cisplatin (40 mg/m^2 IV); repeat every 3 weeks

Potential Problems

- Change in body image
- Dehydration
- Fatigue
- Hypocalcemia
- Hypo-/hyperthyroidism
- Impaired skin integrity
- Infection
- Knowledge deficit
- Obstructed airway
- Radiation thyroiditis
- Sialadenitis

Potential Oncologic Emergencies

- Complete airway obstruction
- Spinal cord compression

Prognosis

- Using Mazzaferri and associates' system, chance of recurrence after 10 years: Stage I, 6.8%; Stage II, 17.4%; Stage III, 36.2%; Stage IV, 50%. Death rates: Stage I, 0.4%; Stage II, 1.3%; Stage III, 9.1%; Stage IV, 60%

Tongue

Epidemiology

- Approximately 5500 new cases per year
- Approximately 1870 deaths per year

Etiology/Risk Factors

- Tobacco use
- Alcohol consumption

Signs and Symptoms

- Aspiration symptoms
- Deep-seated ear pain
- Dysphagia
- Easy bleeding of the mucosal surface
- Erythroplakia
- Garbled, gurgling speech
- Leukoplakia
- Neck mass
- Repeated bleeding from the mouth
- Slow-healing sore
- Unilateral pain

Diagnostic Tests

- Biopsy
- Bone scan
- CBC
- CT
- Chest radiography
- Complete head and neck exam
- Dental consult
- Panendoscopy
- Serum chemistries
- Videoendoscopic exam

Metastatic Sites

- Bone
- Brain
- Liver
- Lung
- Regional lymph nodes

Treatment

- Surgery and radiation therapy are equally effective in treating early-stage (T1, T2) tumors
- For more advanced disease, multimodal therapy with surgery and radiation therapy is used
- Tumors requiring total glossectomy are those that involve the entire tongue or large tumors involving the floor of the mouth and/or the base of the tongue

Potential Problems

- Altered sense of smell
- Anorexia
- Anxiety
- Body image disturbance
- Decreased nutritional intake
- Dental problems
- Dysphagia
- Grieving
- Impaired verbal communication
- Ineffective breathing pattern
- Pain
- Stomatitis
- Taste changes
- Xerostomia

Potential Oncologic Emergencies

- Airway obstruction
- Carotid hemorrhage
- Pneumonia

Prognosis

- 5-year survival rates are variable, depending on the extent of the disease

Ureteral Cancer

Epidemiology
- Approximately 500 cases per year in the United States
- Most frequent histology is transitional cell carcinoma

Etiology/Risk Factors
- Cigarette smoking
- Occupational exposure to chemicals and petroleum
- Phenacetin abuse
- Schistosomiasis
- Chronic inflammation
- Cyclophosphamide exposure

Signs and Symptoms
- Anorexia
- Flank pain
- Hematuria
- Weight loss

Diagnostic Tests
- CT
- IVP
- Retrograde pyelography
- Retrograde urography
- Ureteroscopy
- Urine "cytologies"

Metastatic Sites
- Liver
- Lung
- Regional lymph nodes

Treatment
- Surgical excision is the primary form of treatment
- Systemic chemotherapy—the MVAC regimen (methotrexate, vinblastine, doxorubicin, and cisplatinum)—is usually used for metastatic disease

Potential Problems
- Body image disturbance
- Depression
- Fluid volume excess
- Nutritional deficit
- Pain

Potential Oncologic Emergencies
- Pleural effusions
- Septic shock

Prognosis
- Prognosis varies, depending on stage of disease at time of diagnosis

Uterine Sarcoma

Epidemiology

- 5% of all cancers of the uterus
- Sarcomas arise from the endometrial glands and stroma
- Incidence slightly higher in blacks than in whites

Etiology/Risk Factors

- Pelvic radiation

Signs and Symptoms

- Abdominal mass
- Pelvic pain
- Postmenopausal bleeding
- Uterine bleeding

Diagnostic Tests

- Abdominal and pelvic CT
- Barium enema
- Blood glucose
- CA-125
- CBC
- Chest radiography
- Colonoscopy
- Creatinine level
- Endometrial biopsy
- Fractional D & C
- Liver function tests
- MRI
- PAP smear
- Pelvic examination
- Rectal examination
- Serum electrolytes
- Total bilirubin level
- Vaginal probe ultrasonography

Metastatic Sites

- Abdomen
- Bone
- Brain
- Lung

Treatment

- Hysterectomy, bilateral salphingo-oophorectomy, and pelvic and paraaortic lymph node sampling is the treatment of choice for Stage I disease
- Metastatic disease may require a combination of surgery, radiation therapy, and chemotherapy
- Chemotherapy drugs commonly used for metastatic or recurrent disease include ifosfamide and cisplatin

Potential Problems

- Altered urination
- Body image disturbance
- Nutritional deficit
- Pain

Potential Oncologic Emergencies

- Intestinal obstruction
- Spinal cord compression
- Third space syndrome

Prognosis

- Several factors influence prognosis, including patient age, histology of tumor, depth of myometrial invasion, peritoneal invasion, and presence of distant metastases

Vaginal Cancer

Epidemiology

- 1–2% of all female genital cancers
- 80–90% of vaginal cancers are metastatic

Etiology

- No specific etiologic factors have been identified
- Human papillomavirus may play a role

Signs and Symptoms

- Bladder discomfort
- Constipation
- Dyspareunia
- Leukorrhea
- Pelvic pain
- Postcoital bleeding
- Postmenopausal bleeding
- Tenesmus
- Urinary frequency
- Vaginal spotting

Diagnostic Tests

- Abdominopelvic CT
- Biopsy
- Bone scan
- Chest radiography
- Colposcopy
- Cystoscopy
- Pelvic examination
- Proctoscopy

Metastatic Sites

- Bladder
- Bone
- Breast
- Cervix
- Endometrium
- Kidney
- Liver
- Lungs
- Ovary
- Rectum
- Urethra
- Vulva

Treatment

- Treatment depends on tumor size, location, and clinical stage
- Surgery: radical hysterectomy, vaginectomy, and pelvic lymphadenectomy are sometimes performed for Stage I disease; pelvic exenteration is recommended for recurrent radiation-resistant tumor
- Radiation therapy: treatment of choice using external beam (5000–7500 cGy) with interstitial or intracavitary treatment

Potential Problems

- Altered body image
- Cystitis
- Dyspareunia
- Lymphedema
- Pain
- Proctitis
- Rectal strictures
- Rectovaginal fistulas
- Sexual dysfunction
- Vaginal strictures
- Vesicovaginal fistulas

Potential Oncologic Emergencies

- Intestinal obstruction
- Obstructive uropathy
- Pleural effusions
- Sepsis
- Spinal cord compression

Prognosis

- Survival rates 64–90% for Stage I disease; 29–66% for Stage II; and up to 40% for Stage III or IV.

Vulvar Cancer

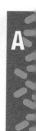

Epidemiology

- Comprises 4% of all cancers of the female genital tract
- Squamous cell carcinoma is the most common type
- Mean age at diagnosis is 65 years
- Disease of postmenopausal women

Etiology/Risk Factors

- Obesity
- Hypertension
- Diabetes mellitus
- Arteriosclerosis
- Early menopause
- Nulliparity
- Human papillomavirus infection
- Cervical cancer
- Syphilis

Signs and Symptoms

- Chronic vulvar pruritus
- Vulvar lump or mass

Diagnostic Tests

- Bone scan
- CT
- Chest radiography
- Cystoscopy
- Liver scan
- Sigmoidoscopy
- Wedge biopsy

Metastatic Sites

- Bladder
- Liver
- Lung
- Pelvic bone
- Rectum
- Regional lymph nodes
- Urethra

Treatment

- Treatment varies, depending on size of tumor and extent of disease
- Stage I lesions may be treated with radical local excision with dissection of the inguinal and femoral lymph nodes
- Stage II vulvar cancer is managed with radical vulvectomy and bilateral inguinofemoral lymphadenectomy
- Radiation therapy may be used preoperatively to shrink tumors or as primary treatment for small anterior tumors
- Chemotherapy using 5-FU or cisplatin to enhance the effectiveness of RT is currently under investigation

Potential Problems

- Altered body image
- Infection
- Lymphangitis
- Lymphedema
- Pain
- Rectovaginal fistulas
- Sexual dysfunction

Potential Oncologic Emergencies

- Intestinal obstruction
- Obstructive uropathy
- Pleural effusions
- Spinal cord compression

Prognosis

- Prognosis correlates with tumor size and lymph node involvement
- Overall survival 47.37%

Wilms' Tumor

Epidemiology

- Most common intraabdominal tumor in children
- 450–500 new cases per year
- Male-female ratio 1:1

Etiology/Risk Factors

- Age 2–5 years
- Associated with hemihypertrophy, aniridia, and genitourinary anomalies
- Inherited in up to 40% of cases
- Can occur in teenagers and adults
- Parental occupational exposure, radiation, drugs, tobacco, and alcohol

Signs and Symptoms

- Early: palpable abdominal mass detected by parent
- Late: fever, abdominal pain, hematuria, and/or hypertension

Diagnostic Tests

- Abdominal ultrasound
- BUN
- CBC
- Chest radiography
- CT
- IVP
- MRI of vena cava
- Serum creatinine
- Skeletal survey
- Urinalysis

Metastatic Sites

- Lung

Treatment

- Surgery: exploration and removal
- Radiation therapy: used to prevent local and regional recurrence of higher-grade tumors
- Adjuvant chemotherapy
  - First-choice agents are dactinomycin (15 μg/kg/day for 5 consecutive days) + vincristine (1.5 mg/m^2/week for 10 weeks, starting on day 7).
  - For higher-grade tumors: adriamycin (20 mg/m^2/day) or cyclophosphamide (10 mg/kg/day) is added to the regimen.

Potential Problems

- Hair loss
- Infection
- Nausea and vomiting
- Peripheral neuropathy
- Renal failure
- Rupture of tumor prior to or during surgery

Potential Oncologic Emergencies

- Bowel obstruction
- Septic shock

Prognosis

- Using the National Wilms' Tumor Study–staging system, 4-year relapse-free survival: favorable-histology Stage I, 89%; Stage II, 88%; Stage III, 78%: Stage IV, 75%; unfavorable histology Stages I to III, 66%; and Stage IV, 55%

Bibliography

Anal Cancer

Carter, P. S. (1993). Anal cancer—current perspectives. *Digestive Diseases, 11*(4–5), 239–251.

Luk, G. D. (1993). Rolling review: Gastrointestinal malignancy. *Alimentary Pharmacology and Therapeutics, 7*(6), 661–677.

Mendenhall, W. M., Sombeck, M. D., Speer, T. W., Marsh, R. D., Carroll, R. R., & Copeland, E. M., 3rd. (1994). Current management of squamous cell carcinoma of the anal canal. *Surgical Oncology, 3*(3), 135–146.

Tarazi, R., & Nelson, R. L. (1994). Anal adenocarcinoma: A comprehensive review. *Seminars in Surgical Oncology, 10*(3), 235–240.

Astrocytoma

Bleehan, N. M., & Ford, J. M. (1993). Radiotherapy, hyperthermia, and photodynamic therapy for central nervous system tumors. *Current Opinion in Oncology, 5*(3), 458–463.

Hoffman, H. J., Soloniuk, D. S., Humphreys, R. P., Drake, J. M., Becker, L. E., De Lima, B. O., & Piatt, J. H., Jr. (1993). Management and outcome of low-grade astrocytomas of the midline in children: A retrospective review. *Neurosurgery, 33*(6), 964–971.

Mangiardi, J. R., & Yodice, P. (1990). Metabolism of the malignant astrocytoma. *Neurosurgery, 26*(1), 1–19.

McCormack, B. M., Miller, D. C., Budzilovich, G. N., Voorhees, G. J., & Ransohoff, J. (1992). Treatment and survival of low-grade astrocytoma in adults—1977–1988. *Neurosurgery, 31*(4), 636–642.

Prados, M. D., Gutin, P. H., Phillips, T. L., Wara, W. M., Larson, D. A., Sneed, P. K., Davis, R. L., Ahn, D. K., Lamborn, K., & Wilson, C. B. Highly anaplastic astrocytoma: A review of 357 patients treated between 1977 and 1989. *International Journal of Radiation Oncology, Biology, Physics, 23*(1), 3–8.

Yates, A. J. (1992). An overview of principles for classifying brain tumors. *Molecular and Chemical Neuropathology, 17*(2), 103–120.

Basal Cell Skin Cancer

Chorun, L., Norris, J. E., & Gupta, M. (1994). Basal cell carcinoma in blacks: A report of 15 cases. *Annals of Plastic Surgery, 33*(1), 90–95.

Kricker, A., Armstrong, B. K., & English, D. R. (1994). Sun exposure and non-melanocytic skin cancer. *Cancer Causes and Control, 5*(4), 367–392.

Lambert, D. R., & Siegle, R. J. (1990). Skin cancer: A review with consideration of treatment options including Mohs micrographic surgery. *Ohio Medicine, 86*(10), 745–747.

Miller, S. J. (1991). Biology of basal cell carcinoma (Part II). *Journal of the American Academy of Dermatology, 24*(2, Pt. 1), 161–175.

Rees, J. (1994). Genetic alterations in non-melanoma skin cancer. *Journal of Investigative Dermatology, 103*(6), 747–750.

Bladder Cancer: Superficial

Batts, C. N. (1992). Adjuvant intravesical therapy for superficial bladder cancer. *Annals of Pharmacotherapy, 26*(10), 1270–1276.

Bouffioux, C. (1991). Intravesical adjuvant treatment in superficial bladder cancer. A review of the question after 15 years of experience with the EORTC GU group. *Scandinavian Journal of Urology and Nephrology, 138*(Suppl.), 167–177.

Friberg, S. (1993). BCG in the treatment of superficial cancer of the bladder: A review. *Medical Oncology and Tumor Pharmacotherapy, 10*(1–2), 31–36.

Hirao, Y., Ozono, S., Momose, H., Okajima, E., Hiramatsu, T., Yoshida, K., Fukushima, S., & Ohashi, Y. (1994). Prospective randomized study of prophylaxis of superficial bladder cancer with epirubicin: The role of a central pathology laboratory. Nara Uro-oncology Research Group. (NUORG). *Cancer Chemotherapy and Pharmacology, 35*(Suppl.), S36–S40.

Jauhiainen, K., & Rintala, E. (1993). Superficial urinary bladder cancer. Results from the Finnbladder studies and a review on instillation treatments. *Annales Chirurgiae et Gynaecologiae, 206*(Suppl.), 31–38.

Kelloff, G. J., Boone, C. W., Malone, W. F., Steele, V. E., & Doody, L. A. (1992). Development of chemopreventive agents for bladder cancer. *Journal of Cellular Biochemistry, 161*(Suppl.), 1–12.

Schalken, J. A., van Moorselaar, R. J., Bringuier, P. P., & Debruyne, F. M. (1992). Critical review of the models to study the biologic progression of bladder cancer. *Seminars in Surgical Oncology, 8*(5), 274–278.

Simoneau, A. R., & Jones, P. A. (1994). Bladder cancer: The molecular progression to invasive disease. *World Journal of Urology, 12*(2), 89–95.

Steg, A., Adjiman, S., & Debre, B. (1992). BCG therapy in superficial bladder tumours—complications and precautions. *European Urology, 21*(Suppl. 2), 35–40.

Witjes, J. A., Kiemeney, L. A., Oosterhof, G. O., & Debruyne, F. M. (1992). Prognostic factors in superficial bladder cancer. A review. *European Urology, 21*(2), 89–97.

Witjes, J. A., Kiemeney, L. A., Schaafsma, H. E., & Debruyn, F. M. (1994). The influence of review pathology on study outcome of a randomized multicentre superficial bladder cancer trial. Members of the Dutch South East Cooperative Urological Group. *British Journal of Urology, 73*(2), 172–176.

Bladder Cancer: Invasive

Cole, C. J., Pollack, A., Zagars, G. K., Dinney, C. P., Swanson, D. A., & von Eschenbach, A. C. (1995). Local control of muscle-invasive bladder cancer: Preoperative radiotherapy and cystectomy versus cystectomy alone. *International Journal of Radiation Oncology, Biology, Physics, 32*(2), 331–340.

Duchesne, G. M. (1994). Radical treatment for primary bladder cancer: Where are we and where do we go from here? A review. *Clinical Oncology (Royal College of Radiologists), 6*(2), 121–126.

Gospodarowicz, M. K., & Warde, P. R. (1993). A critical review of the role of definitive radiation therapy in bladder cancer. *Seminars in Urology, 11*(4), 214–226.

Waehre, H., Ous, S., Klevmark, B., Kvarstein, B., Urnes, T., Ogreid, P., Johansen, T. E., & Fossa, S. D. (1993). A bladder cancer multi-institutional experience with total cystectomy for muscle-invasive bladder cancer. *Cancer, 72*(10), 3044–3051.

Breast Cancer: Noninvasive Disease

Rebner, M., & Raju, U. (1994). Noninvasive breast cancer. *Radiology, 190*(3), 623–631.

Breast Cancer: Early Invasive Disease

Lonning, P. E. (1991). Treatment of early breast cancer with conservation of the breast. A review. *Acta Oncologica, 30*(7), 779–792.

McCormick, B. (1994). Selection criteria for breast conservation. The impact of young and old age and collagen vascular disease. *Cancer, 74*(1, Suppl.), 430–435.

Pisansky, T. M., Halyard, M. Y., Weaver, A. L., Donohue, J. H., Grado, G. L., Grant, C. S., Hartmann, L. C., Ingle, J. N., Schomberg, P. J., & Wold, L. E. (1994). Breast conservation therapy for invasive breast cancer: A review of prior trials and the Mayo Clinic experience. *Mayo Clinic Proceedings, 69*(6), 515–524.

Breast Cancer: Locally Advanced Disease

Ahern, V., Barraclough, B., Bosch, C., Langlands, A., & Boyages, J. (1994). Locally advanced breast cancer: Defining an optimum treatment regimen. *International Journal of Radiation Oncology, Biology, Physics, 28*(4), 867–875.

Hathaway, C. L., Rand, R. P., Moe, R., & Marchioro, T. (1994). Salvage surgery for locally advanced and locally recurrent breast cancer. *Archives of Surgery, 129*(6), 582–587.

Overmoyer, B. A. (1995). Chemotherapy in the management of breast cancer. *Cleveland Clinic Journal of Medicine, 62*(1), 36–50.

Perez, C. A., Graham, M. L., Taylor, M. E., Levy, J. F., Mortimer, J. E., Philpott, G. W., & Kucik, N. A. (1994). Management of locally advanced carcinoma of the breast. I. Noninflammatory. *Cancer, 74*(1, Suppl.), 453–465.

Robertson, J. F., Ellis, I. O., Pearson, D., Elston, C. W., Nicholson, R. I., & Blamey, R. W. (1994). Biological factors of prognostic significance in locally advanced breast cancer. *Breast Cancer Research and Treatment, 29*(3), 259–264.

Burkitt's Lymphoma

Joske, D., & Knecht, H. (1993). Epstein-Barr virus in lymphomas: A review. *Blood Reviews, 7*(4), 215–222.

Kornblau, S. M., Goodacre, A., & Cabanillas, F. (1991). Chromosomal abnormalities in adult non-endemic Burkitt's lymphoma and leukemia: 22 new reports and a review of 148 cases from the literature. *Hematological Oncology, 9*(2), 63–78.

Patton, L. L., McMillan, C. W., & Webster, W. P. (1990). American Burkitt's lymphoma: A 10-year review and case study. *Oral Surgery, Oral Medicine, Oral Pathology, 69*(3), 307–316.

Schuster, V., & Kreth, H. W. (1992). Epstein-Barr virus infection and associated diseases in children. I. Pathogenesis, epidemiology and clinical aspects. *European Journal of Pediatrics, 151*(10), 718–725.

Central Nervous System Lymphoma

Fine, H. A., & Mayer, R. J. (1993). Primary central nervous system lymphoma. *Annals of Internal Medicine, 119*(11), 1093–1104.

Matano, S., Nakamura, S., Ohtake, S., Okumura, H., Okabe, Y., Kanno, M., Takeshima, M., Syouin, K., Nonomura, A., & Yoshida, T. (1994). Primary T cell non-Hodgkin's lymphoma of the central nervous system. Case report and review of the literature. *Acta Haematologica, 91*(3), 158–163.

Remick, S. C., Diamond, C., Migliozzi, J. A., Solis, O., Wagner, H., Jr., Haase, R. F., & Ruckdeschel, J. C. (1990). Primary central nervous system lymphoma in patients with and without the acquired immune deficiency syndrome. A retrospective analysis and review of the literature. *Medicine, 69*(6), 345–360.

Schild, S. E., Wharen, R. E., Jr., Menke, D. M., Folger, W. N., & Colon-Otero, G. (1995). Primary lymphoma of the spinal cord. *Mayo Clinic Proceedings, 70*(3), 256–260.

Selch, M. T., Shimizu, K. T., De Salles, A. F., Sutton, C., & Parker, R. G. (1994). Primary central nervous system lymphoma. Results at the University of California at Los Angeles and review of the literature. *American Journal of Clinical Oncology, 17*(4), 286–293.

Cervical Cancer

Benedet, J. L., Anderson, G. H., & Matisic, J. P. (1992). A comprehensive program for cervical cancer detection and management. *American Journal of Obstetrics and Gynecology, 166*(4), 1254–1259.

Bosch, F. X., Manos, M. M., Munoz, N., Sherman, M., Jansen, A. M., Peto, J., Schiffman, M. H., Moreno, V., Kurman, R., & Shah, K. V. (1995). Prevalence of human papillomavirus in cervical cancer: A worldwide perspective. International biological study on cervical cancer (IBSCC) Study Group. *Journal of the National Cancer Institute, 87*(11), 796–802.

Friedlander, M., de Souza, P., & Segelov, E. (1992). Risk factors, epidemiology, screening, and prognostic factors in female genital cancer. *Current Opinion in Oncology, 4*(5), 913–922.

Gotlieb, W. H., & Berek, J. S. (1994). Advances in the biology of gynecologic cancer. *Current Opinion in Oncology, 6*(5), 513–518.

Inman, G. J., Cook, I. D., & Lau, R. K. (1993). Human papillomaviruses, tumour suppressor genes and cervical cancer. *International Journal of STD and AIDS, 4*(3), 128–134.

Jones, W. B. (1993). New approaches to high-risk cervical cancer. Advanced cervical cancer. *Cancer, 71*(4, Suppl.), 1451–1491.

Krumm, S., & Lamberti, J. (1993). Changes in sexual behavior following radiation therapy for cervical cancer. *Journal of Psychosomatic Obstetrics and Gynaecology, 14*(1), 51–63.

Lanciano, R. M., & Corn, B. W. (1992). Radiotherapy for gynecologic malignancies. *Current Opinion in Oncology, 4*(5), 930–938.

Orr, J. W., Jr., & Holloway, R. W. (1991). Surgical aspects of cervical cancer. *Surgical Clinics of North America, 71*(5), 1067–1083.

Park, R. C., & Thigpen, J. T. (1993). Chemotherapy in advanced and recurrent cervical cancer. A review. *Cancer, 71*(4, Suppl.), 1446–1450.

Potischman, N. (1993). Nutritional epidemiology of cervical neoplasia. *Journal of Nutrition, 123*(2, Suppl.), 424–429.

Robert, M. E., & Fu, Y. S. (1990). Squamous cell carcinoma of the uterine cervix—a review with emphasis on prognostic factors and unusual variants. *Seminars in Diagnostic Pathology, 7*(3), 173–189.

Colon Cancer

de Braud, F., Bajetta, E., Di Bartolomeo, M., & Colleoni, M. (1992). Adjuvant chemotherapy for cancer of gastrointestinal tract: A critical review. *Tumori, 78*(4), 228–234.

Ferrucci, J. T. (1993). Screening for colon cancer: Controversies and recommendations. *Radiologic Clinics of North America, 31*(6), 1189–1195.

Hough, D. M., Malone, D. E., Rawlinson, J., De Gara, C. J., Moote, D. J., Irvine, E. J., Somers, S., & Stevenson, G. W. (1994). Colon cancer detection: An algorithm using endoscopy and barium enema. *Clinical Radiology, 49*(3), 170–175.

Lopez, M. (1994). Adjuvant therapy of colorectal cancer. *Diseases of the Colon and Rectum, 37*(2, Suppl.), S86–S91.

Potter, J. D., Slattery, M. L., Bostick, R. M., & Gapstur, S. M. (1993). Colon cancer: A review of the epidemiology. *Epidemiologic Reviews, 15*(2), 499–545.

Wayne, M. S., Cath, A., & Pamies, R. J. (1995). Colorectal cancer. A practical review for the primary care physician. *Archives of Family Medicine, 4*(4), 357–366.

Cutaneous Lymphoma

Bunn, P. A., Jr., Hoffman, S. J., Norris, D., Golitz, L. E., & Aeling, J. L. (1994). Systemic therapy of cutaneous T-cell lymphomas (mycosis fungoides and the Sezary syndrome). *Annals of Internal Medicine, 121*(8), 592–602.

Kerrigan, K. (1994). Lymphomatoid papulosis: A model of lymphomagenesis. *Dermatology Nursing, 6*(6), 429–435.

Rijaarsdam, J. U., & Willemze, R. (1994). Primary cutaneous B-cell lymphomas. *Leukemia and Lymphoma, 14*(3–4), 213–218.

Slater, D. N. (1994). Review of investigative diagnostic techniques for cutaneous lymphoma. *Seminars in Dermatology, 13*(3), 166–171.

Wolfe, J. T., Lessin, S. R., Singh, A. H., & Rook, A. H. (1994). Review of immunomodulation by photopheresis: Treatment of cutaneous T-cell lymphoma, autoimmune disease, and allograft rejection. *Artificial Organs, 18*(12), 888–897.

Zackheim, H. S. (1994). Treatment of cutaneous T-cell lymphoma. *Seminars in Dermatology, 13*(3), 207–215.

Zemtsov, A., & Camisa C. (1990). Treatment of primary cutaneous B cell lymphoma with local radiotherapy. *Cutis, 45*(6), 435–438.

Endometrial Cancer

Friedlander, M., de Souza, P., & Segelov, E. (1992). Risk factors, epidemiology, screening, and prognostic factors in female genital cancer. *Current Opinion in Oncology, 4*(5), 913–922.

Grady, D., Gebretsadik, T., Kerlikowske, K., Ernster, V., & Petitti D. (1995). Hormone replacement therapy and endometrial cancer risk: A meta-analysis. *Obstetrics and Gynecology, 85*(2), 304–313.

Lanciano, R. M., & Corn, B. W. (1992). Radiotherapy for gynecologic malignancies. *Current Opinion in Oncology, 4*(5), 930–938.

Levenback, C. (1994). Gynecologic oncology: A review for ET nurses. *Journal of Wound, Ostomy, and Continence Nursing, 21*(4), 141–148.

Photopulos, G. J. (1994). Surgicopathologic staging of endometrial adenocarcinoma. *Current Opinion in Obstetrics and Gynecology, 6*(1), 92–97.

Savino, L., Baldini, B., Susini, T., Pulli, F., Antignani, L., & Massi, G. B. (1992). GnRH analogs in gynecological oncology: A review. *Journal of Chemotherapy, 4*(5), 312–320.

Shumsky, A. G., Stuart, G. C., Brasher, P. M., Nation, J. G., Robertson, D. I., & Sangkarat, S. (1994). An evaluation of routine follow-up of patients treated for endometrial carcinoma. *Gynecologic Oncology, 55*(2), 229–233.

Esophageal Cancer

Fagerberg, J., Stockeld D., & Lewensohn, R. (1994). Combined treatment modalities in esophageal cancer. Should chemotherapy be included? *Acta Oncologica, 33*(4), 439–450.

Maehara, Y., Kuwano, H., Kitamura, K., Matsuda, H., & Sugimachi, K. (1992). Hyperthermochemoradiotherapy for esophageal cancer. *Anticancer Research, 12*(3), 805–810.

Mirvish, S. S. (1995). Role of N-nitroso compounds (NOC) and N-nitrosation in etiology of gastric, esophageal, nasopharyngeal and bladder cancer and contribution to cancer of known exposures to NOC. *Cancer Letters, 93*(1), 17–48.

Pera, M., Cameron, A. J., Trastek, V. F., Carpenter, H. A., & Zinsmeister, A. R. Increasing incidence of adenocarcinoma of the esophagus and esophagogastric junction. *Gastroenterology, 104*(2), 510–513.

Stemmermann, G., Heffelfinger, S. C., Noffsinger, A., Hui, Y. Z., Miller, M. A., & Fenoglio-Preiser,

C. M. (1994). The molecular biology of esophageal and gastric cancer and their precursors: Oncogenes, tumor suppressor genes, and growth factors. *Human Pathology, 25*(10), 968–981.

Viswanathan, V., & Fleischer, D. (1995). Esophageal cancer. Diagnosis and treatment. *Gastroenterologist, 3*(1), 3–13.

Glioma

Janus, T. J., Kyritsis, A. P., Forman, A. D., & Levin, V. A. (1992). Biology and treatment of gliomas. *Annals of Oncology, 3*(6), 423–433.

Kornblith, P. K., Welch, W. C., & Bradley, M. K. (1993). The future of therapy for glioblastoma. *Surgical Neurology, 39*(6), 538–543.

Linskey, M. E., & Gilbert, M. R. (1995). Glial differentiation: A review with implications for new directions in neuro-oncology. *Neurosurgery, 36*(1), 1–21.

Maria, B. L., Eskin, T. A., & Quisling, R. G. (1993). Brainstem and other malignant gliomas: II. Possible mechanisms of brain infiltration by tumor cells. *Journal of Child Neurology, 8*(4), 292–305.

Miller, D. C., Lang, F. F., & Epstein, F. J. (1993). Central nervous system gangliogliomas. Part 1: Pathology. *Journal of Neurosurgery, 79*(6), 859–866.

Salvati, M., Puzzilli, F., Bristot, R., & Cervoni, L. (1994). Post-radiation gliomas. *Tumori, 80*(3), 220–223.

Weingart, J., & Brem, H. (1992). Biology and therapy of glial tumors. *Current Opinion in Neurology and Neurosurgery, 5*(6), 808–812.

Hepatocellular Cancer

Arbaje, Y. M., & Carbone, P. P. (1994). Hepatocellular carcinoma in the very elderly: To treat or not to treat? *Medical and Pediatric Oncology, 22*(2), 84–87.

Keeffe, E. B., & Esquivel, C. O. (1993). Controversies in patient selection for liver transplantation. *Western Journal of Medicine, 159*(5), 586–593.

Yuki, K., Hirohashi, S., Sakamoto, M., Kanai, T., & Shimosato, Y. (1990). Growth and spread of hepatocellular carcinoma. A review of 240 consecutive autopsy cases. *Cancer, 66*(10), 2174–2179.

Hodgkin's Disease

Butler, J. J., & Pugh, W. C. (1993). Review of Hodgkin's disease. *Hematologic Pathology, 7*(2), 59–77.

Fleury, J., Legros, M., Cure, H., Tortochaux, J., Condat, P., Dionet, C., Travade, P., Belembaogo, E., Tavernier, F, & Kwiatkowski, F. (1994). The hematopoietic stem cell transplantation in Hodgkin's disease: Questions and controversies. *Leukemia and Lymphoma, 15*(5–6), 419–432.

Samoszuk, M., & Ramzi, E. (1993). IgE, Reed-Sternberg cells, and eosinophilia in Hodgkin's disease. *Leukemia and Lymphoma, 9*(4–5), 315–319.

Straus, D. J. (1993). Treatment of early stage Hodgkin's disease. *Blood Reviews, 7*(1), 34–42.

Laryngeal Cancer

McCaffrey, T. V. (1992). Head and neck cancer surgery. *Current Opinion in Oncology, 4*(3), 499–503.

Morris, M. R., Canonico, D., & Blank, C. (1994). A critical review of radiotherapy in the management of T1 glottic carcinoma. *American Journal of Otolaryngology, 15*(4), 276–280.

Panje, W. R., Namon, A. J., Vokes, E., Haraf, D. J., & Weichselbaum, R. R. (1995). Surgical management of the head and neck cancer patient following concomitant multimodality therapy. *Laryngoscope, 105*(1), 97–101.

al-Sarraf, M., & Hussein, M. (1995). Head and neck cancer: Present status and future prospects of adjuvant chemotherapy. *Cancer Investigation, 13*(1), 41–53.

Suzuki, H., Hasegawa, T., Sano, R., & Kim, Y. (1994). Results of treatment of laryngeal cancer. *Acta Oto-Laryngologica (Stockholm), 511*(Suppl.), 186–191.

Leukemia: Acute Lymphoblastic

Bleyer, W. A. (1990). Acute lymphoblastic leukemia in children. Advances and prospectus. *Cancer, 65*(3, Suppl.), 689–695.

Borowitz, M. J. (1990). Immunologic markers in childhood acute lymphoblastic leukemia. *Hematology/Oncology Clinics of North America, 4*(4), 743–765.

Botti, A. C., & Verma, R. S. (1990). The molecular biology of acute lymphoblastic leukemia. *Anticancer Research, 10*(2B), 519–525.

Chopra, R., & Goldstone, A. H. (1992). Modern trends in bone marrow transplantation for acute myeloid and acute lymphoblastic leukemia. *Current Opinion in Oncology, 4*(2), 247–258.

Kumar, L. (1994). Leukemia: Management of relapse after allogeneic bone marrow transplantation. *Journal of Clinical Oncology, 12*(8), 1710–1717.

Taylor, P. R., Reid, M. M., & Proctor, S. J. Acute lymphoblastic leukaemia in the elderly. *Leukemia and Lymphoma, 13*(5–6), 373–380.

Leukemia: Acute Myelogenous

Bassan, R., & Barbui, T. (1995). Remission induction therapy for adults with acute myelogenous leukemia: Towards the ICE age? *Haematologica, 80*(1), 82–90.

Berman, E. (1992). New drugs in acute myelogenous leukemia: A review. *Journal of Clinical Pharmacology, 32*(4), 296–309.

Dann, E. J., Gillis, S., & Rowe, J. M. (1995). Late relapse following autologous bone marrow transplantation for acute myelogenous leukemia: Case report and review of the literature. *Leukemia, 9*(6), 1072–1074.

Mastrianni, D. M., Tung, N. M., & Tenen, D. G. (1992). Acute myelogenous leukemia: Current treatment and future directions. *American Journal of Medicine, 92*(3), 286–295.

Vogler, W. R. (1992). Strategies in the treatment of acute myelogenous leukemia. *Leukemia Research, 16*(12), 1143–1153.

Yeager, K. A., & Miaskowski, C. (1994). Advances in understanding the mechanisms and management of acute myelogenous leukemia. *Oncology Nursing Forum, 21*(3), 541–548.

Zittoun, R. (1992). Chemotherapy of acute myelogenous leukemia. A review. *Leukemia, 6*(Suppl. 2), 36–38.

Leukemia: Chronic Lymphocytic

Bandini, G., Michallet, M., Rosti, G., & Tura, S. (1991). Bone marrow transplantation for chronic lymphocytic leukemia. *Bone Marrow Transplantation, 7*(4), 251–253.

Dicato, M., Chapel, H., Gamm, H., Lee, M., Ries, F., Marichal, S., Wirth, C., Griffith, H., & Brennan, V. (1991). Use of intravenous immunoglobulin in chronic lymphocytic leukemia. A brief review. *Cancer, 68*(6, Suppl.), 1437–1439.

Faguet, G. B. (1994). Chronic lymphocytic leukemia: An updated review. *Journal of Clinical Oncology, 12*(9), 1974–1990.

Foon, K. A., Rai, K. R., & Gale, R. P. (1990). Chronic lymphocytic leukemia: New insights into biology and therapy. *Annals of Internal Medicine, 113*(7), 525–539.

Leukemia: Chronic Myelogenous

Aulitzky, W. E., Peschel, C., Schneller, F., & Huber, C. (1995). Biotherapy of chronic myelogenous leukemia. *Annals of Hematology, 70*(3), 113–120.

Gale, R. P., & Butturini, A. (1993). Recent progress in understanding chronic myelogenous leukemia. *Leukemia and Lymphoma, 11*(Suppl. 1), 3–5.

Leukemia: Hairy Cell Leukemia

Frassoldati, A., Lamparelli, T., Federico, M., Annino, L., Capnist, G., Pagnucco, G., Dini, E., Resegotti, L., Damasio, E. E., & Silingardi, V. (1994). Hairy cell leukemia: A clinical review based on 725 cases of the Italian Cooperative Group (ICGHCL). Italian Cooperative Group for Hairy Cell Leukemia. *Leukemia and Lymphoma, 13*(3–4), 307–316.

Golomb, H. M., & Ellis, E. (1991). Treatment options for hairy-cell leukemia. *Seminars in Oncology, 18*(5, Suppl. 7), 7–11.

Hjelle, B. (1991). (Human T-cell leukemia/lymphoma viruses. Life cycle, pathogenicity, epidemiology, and diagnosis. *Archives of Pathology and Laboratory Medicine, 115*(5), 440–450.

Jaiyesimi, I. A., Kantarjian, H. M., & Estey, E. H. (1993). Advances in therapy for hairy cell leukemia. A review. *Cancer, 72*(1), 5–16.

Kurzrock, R., Talpaz, M., & Gutterman, J. U. (1991). Hairy cell leukemia: Review of treatment. *British Journal of Haematology, 79*(Suppl. 1), 17–20.

Vedantham, S., Gamliel, H., & Golomb, H. M. (1992). Mechanism of interferon action in hairy cell leukemia: A model of effective cancer biotherapy. *Cancer Research, 52*(5), 1056–1066.

Lung Cancer: Large Cell

Jaklitsch, M. T., Strauss, G. M., & Sugarbaker, D. J. (1993). Neoadjuvant and adjuvant therapy in the management of locally advanced non–small-cell lung cancer. *World Journal of Surgery, 17*(6), 729–734.

Lederle, F. A., & Niewoehner, D. E. (1994). Lung cancer surgery. A critical review of the evidence. *Archives of Internal Medicine, 154*(21), 2397–2400.

Lilenbaum, R. C., & Green, M. R. (1993). Novel chemotherapeutic agents in the treatment of non–small-cell lung cancer. *Journal of Clinical Oncology, 11*(7), 1391–1402.

Murren, J. R., & Buzaid, A. C. (1993). Chemotherapy and radiation for the treatment of non–small-cell lung cancer. A critical review. *Clinics in Chest Medicine, 14*(1), 161–171.

Strauss, G. M., Kwiatkowski, D. J., Harpole, D. H., Lynch, T. J., Skarin, A. T., & Sugarbaker, D. J. (1995). Molecular and pathologic markers in stage I non–small-cell carcinoma of the lung.

Journal of the Clinical Oncology, 13(5), 1265–1279.

Lung Cancer: Small Cell

Glover, J., & Miaskowski, C. (1994). Small cell lung cancer: Pathophysiologic mechanisms and nursing implications. Oncology Nursing Forum, 21(1), 87–95.

Hirsch, F. R., Dombernowsky, P., & Hansen, H. H. (1994). Treatment of small cell lung cancer: The Copenhagen experience. Anticancer Research, 14(1B), 317–319.

Niklinski, J., & Furman, M. (1995). Clinical tumour markers in lung cancer. European Journal of Cancer Prevention, 4(2), 129–138.

Shepherd, F. A., Amdemichael, E., Evans, W. K., Chalvardjian, P., Hogg-Johnson, S., Coates, R., & Paul, K. (1994). Treatment of small cell lung cancer in the elderly. Journal of the American Geriatrics Society, 42(1), 64–70.

Splinter, T. A. (1992). Therapy for small cell and non–small cell lung cancer. Current Opinion in Oncology, 4(2), 315–322.

Stahel, R. A. (1994). Biology of lung cancer. Lung Cancer, 10(Suppl. 1), S59–S65.

Trillet-Lenoir, V. N. (1995). The role of hematopoietic growth factors in small cell lung cancer: A review. Cancer Treatment and Research, 72, 273–292.

Lymphocytic Lymphoma

Shivdasani, R. A., Hess, J. L., Skarin, A. T., & Pinkus, G. S. (1993). Intermediate lymphocytic lymphoma: Clinical and pathologic features of a recently characterized subtype of non-Hodgkin's lymphoma. Journal of Clinical Oncology, 11(4), 802–811.

Malignant Melanoma

Evans, G. R., & Manson, P. N. (1994). Review and current perspectives of cutaneous malignant melanoma. Journal of the American College of Surgeons, 178(5), 523–540.

Evans, R. A. (1994). Review and current perspectives of cutaneous malignant melanoma. Journal of the American College of Surgeons, 179(6), 764–767.

Joob, A. W., Haines, G. K., 3rd, Kies, M. S., & Shields, T. W. (1995). Primary malignant melanoma of the esophagus. Annals of Thoracic Surgery, 60(1), 217–222.

Medulloblastoma

Becker, R. L., Becker, A. D., & Sobel, D. F. (1995). Adult medulloblastoma: Review of 13 cases with emphasis on MRI. Neuroradiology, 37(2), 104–108.

Frost, P. J., Laperriere, N. J., Wong, C. S., Milosevic, M. F., Simpson, W. J., & Pintilie, M. (1995). Medulloblastoma in adults. International Journal of Radiation Oncology, Biology, Physics, 32(4), 951–957.

Tomlinson, F. H., Scheithauer, B. W., Meyer, F. B., Smithson, W. A., Shaw, E. G., Miller, G. M., & Groover, R. V. (1992). Medulloblastoma: I. Clinical, diagnostic, and therapeutic overview. Journal of Child Neurology, 7(2), 142–155.

Multiple Myeloma

Barker, H. F., Ball, J., Drew, M., & Franklin, I. M. (1993). Multiple myeloma: The biology of malignant plasma cells. Blood Reviews, 7(1), 19–23.

Fermand, J. P., & Brouet, J. C. (1995). Marrow transplantation for myeloma. Annual Review of Medicine, 46, 299–307.

Huang, Y. W., & Vitetta, E. S. (1995). Immunotherapy of multiple myeloma. Stem Cells, 13(2), 123–134.

Hussein, M. (1994). Multiple myeloma: An overview of diagnosis and management. Cleveland Clinic Journal of Medicine, 61(4), 285–298.

Oken, M. M. (1994). Standard treatment of multiple myeloma. Mayo Clinic Proceedings, 69(8), 781–786.

Nasopharyngeal Cancer

Altun, M., Fandi, A., Dupuis, O., Cvitkovic, E., Krajina, Z., & Eschwege, F. Undifferentiated nasopharyngeal cancer (UCNT): Current diagnostic and therapeutic aspects. International Journal of Radiation Oncology, Biology, Physics, 32(3), 859–877.

Choo, R., & Tannock, I. (1991). Chemotherapy for recurrent or metastatic carcinoma of the nasopharynx. A review of the Princess Margaret Hospital experience. Cancer, 68(10), 2120–2124.

Mirvish, S. S. (1995). Role of N-nitroso compounds (NOC) and N-nitrosation in etiology of gastric, esophageal, nasopharyngeal and bladder cancer and contribution to cancer of known exposures to NOC. Cancer Letters, 93(1), 17–48.

Neuroblastoma

Brodeur, G. M., Pritchard, J., Berthold, F., Carlsen, N. L., Castel, V., Castleberry, R. P., De Bernardi, B., Evans, A. E., Favrot, M., & Hedborg, F. (1993). Revisions of the international criteria for neuroblastoma diagnosis, staging, and response to treatment. Journal of Clinical Oncology, 11(8), 1466–1477.

Di Caro, A., Bostrom, B., Moss, T. J., Neglia, J., Ramsay, N. K., Smith, J., & Sasky, L. C. (1994). Autologous peripheral blood cell transplantation in the treatment of advanced neuroblastoma. American Journal of Pediatric Hematology/Oncology, 16(3), 200–206.

Castleberry, R. P. (1992). Clinical and biologic features in the prognosis and treatment of neuroblastoma. Current Opinion in Oncology, 4(1), 116–123.

Cohen, M. D., Auringer, S. T., Grosfeld, J. L., Galliani, C. A., & Heerema, N. A. (1993). Multifocal primary neuroblastoma. Pediatric Radiology, 23(6), 463–466.

Ishiguro, Y., Iio, K., Seo, T., Nagaya, M., & Ito, T. (1994). Bilateral adrenal neuroblastoma. European Journal of Pediatric Surgery, 4(1), 37–39.

Kiely, E. M. (1994). The surgical challenge of neuroblastoma. Journal of Pediatric Surgery, 29(2), 128–133.

Oropharyngeal Cancer

Wang, C. C., Montgomery, W., & Efird, J. (1995). Local control of oropharyngeal carcinoma by irradiation alone. Laryngoscope, 105(5, Pt. 1), 529–533.

Osteogenic Sarcoma

Carter, S. R., Grimer, R. J., & Sneath, R. S. (1991). A review of 13-years experience of osteosarcoma. Clinical Orthopaedics and Related Research, 270, 45–51.

Meyers, P. A., Heller, G., & Healey, J. (1992). Retrospective review of neoadjuvant chemotherapy for osteogenic sarcoma. Journal of the National Cancer Institute, 84(3), 202–204.

Ovarian Cancer

Abel, U. (1992). Chemotherapy of advanced epithelial cancer—a critical review. Biomedicine and Pharmacotherapy, 46(10), 439–452.

Blend, M. J., & Ostrowski, G. J. (1994). Recent advances in the detection of ovarian cancer: A review. Journal of the American Osteopathic Association, 94(4), 305–318.

Dembo, A. J. (1992). Epithelial ovarian cancer: The role of radiotherapy. International Journal of Radiation Oncology, Biology, Physics, 22(5), 835–845.

Farias-Eisner, R., Kim, Y. B., & Berek, J. S. (1994). Surgical management of ovarian cancer. Seminars in Surgical Oncology, 10(4), 268–275.

Herbst, A. L. (1994). The epidemiology of ovarian carcinoma and the current status of tumor markers to detect disease. American Journal of Obstetrics and Gynecology, 170(4), 1099–1105.

Omura, G. A., & Siller, B. S. (1994). Primary chemotherapy of epithelial ovarian carcinoma. Seminars in Surgical Oncology, 10(4), 283–287.

Rubin, S. C., Wong, G. Y., Curtin, J. P., Barakat, R. R., Hakes, T. B., & Hoskins, W. J. (1993). Platinum-based chemotherapy of high-risk stage I epithelial ovarian cancer following comprehensive surgical staging. Obstetrics and Gynecology, 82(1), 143–147.

Shoham, Z. (1994). Epidemiology, etiology, and fertility drugs in ovarian epithelial carcinoma: Where are we today? Fertility and Sterility, 62(3), 433–448.

Pancreatic Cancer

Eskelinen, M., & Lipponen, P. (1992). A review of prognostic factors in human pancreatic adenocarcinoma. Cancer Detection and Prevention, 16(5–6), 287–295.

Evans, D. B., Rich, T. A., Byrd, D. R., & Ames, F. C. (1991). Adenocarcinoma of the pancreas: Current management of resectable and locally advanced disease. Southern Medical Journal, 84(5), 566–570.

Foutch, P. G. (1994). A diagnostic approach to pancreatic cancer. Digestive Diseases, 12(3), 129–138.

Ho, J. J., & Kim, Y. S. (1994). Serological pancreatic tumor markers and the MUC1 apomucin. Pancreas, 9(6), 674–691.

Moesta, K. T., Schlag, P., Douglass, H. O., Jr., & Mang, T. S. (1995). Evaluating the role of photodynamic therapy in the management of pancreatic cancer. Lasers in Surgery and Medicine, 16(1), 84–92.

Poston, G. J., Gillespie, J., & Guillou, P. J. (1991). Biology of pancreatic cancer. Gut, 32(7), 800–812.

Watanapa, P., & Williamson, R. C. (1992). Surgical palliation for pancreatic cancer: Developments during the past two decades. British Journal of Surgery, 79(1), 8–20.

Wils, J. A. (1991). Chemotherapy in pancreatic cancer: A rational pursuit? Anti-Cancer Drugs, 2(1), 3–10.

Prostate Cancer

Austenfeld, M. S., Thompson, I. M., Jr., & Middleton, R. G. (1994). Meta-analysis of the literature: Guideline development for prostate cancer treatment. American Urological Association Prostate Cancer Guideline Panel. *Journal of Urology, 152*(5, Pt. 2), 1866–1869.

Geller, J. (1995). Clinical review: 67: Approach to chemoprevention of prostate cancer. *Journal of Clinical Endocrinology and Metabolism, 80*(3), 717–719.

Gerber, G. S. (1994). Conservative approach to the management of prostate cancer. A critical review. *European Urology, 26*(4), 271–275.

Held, J. L., Osborne, D. M., Volpe, H., & Waldman, A. R. (1994). Cancer of the prostate: Treatment and nursing implications. *Oncology Nursing Forum, 21*(9), 1517–1529.

Joensuu, T. K., Blomqvist, C. P., & Kajanti, M. J. (1995). Primary radiation therapy in the treatment of localized prostatic cancer. *Acta Oncologica, 34*(2), 183–191.

Netto, G. J., & Humphrey, P. A. (1994). Molecular biologic aspects of human prostatic carcinoma. *American Journal of Clinical Pathology, 102*(4, Suppl. 1), S57–S64.

Pienta, K. J., & Esper, P. S. (1993). Risk factors for prostate cancer. *Annals of Internal Medicine, 118*(10), 793–803.

Rectal Cancer

Baigrie, R. J., & Berry, A. R. (1994). Management of advanced rectal cancer. *British Journal of Surgery, 81*(3), 343–352.

Forman, W. B. (1994). The role of chemotherapy and adjuvant therapy in the management of colorectal cancer. *Cancer, 74*(7, Suppl.), 2151–2153.

Di Matteo, G., Mascagni, D., Lentini, A., Tarroni, D., & Filippini, A. (1994). Advances in rectal cancer surgery. *Diseases of the Colon and Rectum, 37*(2, Suppl.), S50–S53.

Herrera, L., & Brown, M. T. (1994). Prognostic profile in rectal cancer. *Diseases of the Colon and Rectum, 37*(2, Suppl.), S1–S5.

Lopez, M. (1994). Adjuvant therapy of colorectal cancer. *Diseases of the Colon and Rectum, 37*(2, Suppl.), S86–S91.

Myerson, R. J., Michalski, J. M., King, M. L., Birnbaum, E., Fleshman, J., Fry, R., Kodner, I., Lacey, D., & Lockett, M. A. (1995). Adjuvant radiation therapy for rectal carcinoma: Predictors of outcome. *International Journal of Radiation Oncology, Biology, Physics, 32*(1), 41–50.

Tarazi, R., & Nelson, R. L. (1994). Anal adenocarcinoma: A comprehensive review. *Seminars in Surgical Oncology, 10*(3), 235–240.

Renal Cell Cancer

Guinan, P., Saffrin, R., Stuhldreher, D., Frank, W., & Rubenstein, M. (1994). Renal cell carcinoma: Comparison of the TNM and Robson stage groupings. *Journal of Surgical Oncology, 59*(3), 186–189.

Stadler, W., & Vogelzang, N. J. (1993). Human renal cancer carcinogenesis: A review of recent advances. *Annals of Oncology, 4*(6), 451–462.

Sarcoma: Soft Tissue

Kraybill, W. G., Emami, B., & Lyss, A. P. (1991). Management of soft tissue sarcomas of the extremities. *Surgery, 109*(3, Pt. 1), 233–235.

Marcus, S. G., Merino, M. J., Glatstein, E., DeLaney, T. F., Steinberg, S. M., Rosenberg, S. A., & Yang, J. C. (1993). Long-term outcome in 87 patients with low-grade soft-tissue sarcoma. *Archives of Surgery, 128*(12), 1336–1343.

Munk, P. L., Poon, P. Y., Chhem, R. K., & Janzen, D. L. (1994). Imaging of soft-tissue sarcomas. *Canadian Association of Radiologists Journal, 45*(6), 438–446.

Small Intestine Cancer: Adenocarcinoma

Bauer, R. L., Palmer, M. L., Bauer, A. M., Nava, H. R., & Douglass, H. O., Jr. (1994). Adenocarcinoma of the small intestine: 21-year review of diagnosis, treatment, and prognosis. *Annals of Surgical Oncology, 1*(3), 183–188.

Frost, D. B., Mercado, P. D., & Tyrell, J. S. (1994). Small bowel cancer: A 30-year review. *Annals of Surgical Oncology, 1*(4), 290–295.

Di Sario, J. A., Burt, R. W., Vargas, H., & McWhorter, W. P. (1994). Small bowel cancer: Epidemiological and clinical characteristics from a population-based registry. *American Journal of Gastroenterology, 89*(5), 699–701.

Small Intestine Cancer: Lymphoma

Varghese, C., Jose, C. C., Subhashini, J., & Roul, R. K. (1992). Primary small intestinal lymphoma. *Oncology, 49*(5), 340–342.

Small Intestine Cancer: Sarcoma

Horowitz, J., Spellman, J. E., Jr., Driscoll, D. L., Velez, A. F., & Karakousis, C. P. (1995). An institutional review of sarcomas of the large and small intestine. *Journal of the American College of Surgeons, 180*(4), 465–471.

Stomach Cancer

Antonioli, D. A. (1994). Precursors of gastric carcinoma: A critical review with a brief description of early (curable) gastric cancer. *Human Pathology, 25*(10), 994–1005.

Arak, A., & Kull, K. (1994). Factors influencing survival of patients after radical surgery for gastric cancer. A regional study of 406 patients over a 10-year period. *Acta Oncologica, 33*(8), 913–920.

Haglund, U., Wollert, S., & Gustavsson, S. (1990). Gastric cancer. A selective clinical review. *Acta Chirurgica Scandinavica, 156*(1), 99–104.

Hermans, J., Bonenkamp, J. J., Boon, M. C., Bunt, A. M., Ohyama, S., Sasako, M., & Van de Velde, C. J. (1993). Adjuvant therapy after curative resection for gastric cancer: Meta-analysis of randomized trials. *Journal of Clinical Oncology, 11*(8), 1441–1447.

Stemmermann, G., Heffelfinger, S. C., Noffsinger, A., Hui, Y. Z., Miller, M. A., & Fenoglio-Preiser, C. M. (1994). The molecular biology of esophageal and gastric cancer and their precursors: Oncogenes, tumor suppressor genes, and growth factors. *Human Pathology, 25*(10), 968–981.

Tabuenca, A. D., Aitken, D. R., Ihde, J. K., Smith, J., & Garberoglio, C. (1993). Factors influencing survival in advanced gastric cancer. *American Surgeon, 59*(12), 855–859.

Takeda, J., Koufuji, K., Kodama, I., Tsuji, Y., Yokoyama, T., Kawabata, S., Suematsu, T., & Kakegawa, T. (1994). Total gastrectomy for gastric cancer: 12-year data and review of the effect of performing lymphadenectomy. *Kurume Medical Journal, 41*(1), 15–21.

Testicular Cancer

Baniel, J., Foster, R. S., Gonin, R., Messemer, J. E., Donohue, J. P., & Einhon, L. H. (1995). Late relapse of testicular cancer. *Journal of Clinical Oncology, 13*(5), 1170–1176.

Javadpour, N. (1992). Current status of tumor markers in testicular cancer. A practical review. *European Urology, 21*(Suppl. 1), 34–36.

Moul, J. W., Schanne, F. J., Thompson, I. M., Frazier, H. A., Peretsman, S. A., Wettlaufer, J. N., Rozanski, T. A., Stack, R. S., Kreder, K. J., & Hoffman, K. J. (1994). Testicular cancer in blacks. A multicenter experience. *Cancer, 73*(2), 388–393.

Rosella, J. D. (1994). Testicular cancer health education: An integrative review. *Journal of Advanced Nursing, 20*(4), 666–671.

Stone, J. M., Sandeman, T. F., Ironside, P., Cruickshank, D. G., & Matthews, J. P. (1992). Time trends in accuracy of classification of testicular tumours, with clinical and epidemiological implications. *British Journal of Cancer, 66*(2), 396–401.

Williams, S. D., & Roth, B. J. (1992). Chemotherapy of testis cancer: A review. *International Journal of Radiation Oncology, Biology, Physics, 22*(1), 213–217.

Thyroid Cancer

Baker, K. H., & Feldman, J. E. (1993). Thyroid cancer: A review. *Oncology Nursing Forum, 20*(1), 95–104.

Clark, O. H., & Duh, Q. Y. (1991). Thyroid cancer. *Medical Clinics of North America, 75*(1), 211–234.

Franceschi, S., Boyle, P., Maisonneuve, P., La Vecchia, C., Burt, A. D., Kerr, D. J., & MacFarlane, G. J. (1993). The epidemiology of thyroid carcinoma. *Critical Reviews in Oncogenesis, 4*(1), 25–52.

Hennen, G. (1994). Cancer of the thyroid— explorations of clinical biology. *Acta Chirurgica Belgica, 94*(1), 30–32.

O'Doherty, M. J., Nunan, T. O., & Croft, D. N. (1993). Radionuclides and therapy of thyroid cancer. *Nuclear Medicine Communications, 14*(9), 736–755.

Tongue Cancer

Sarkaria, J. N., & Harari, P. M. (1994). Oral tongue cancer in young adults less than 40 years of age: Rationale for aggressive therapy. *Head and Neck, 16*(2), 107–111.

Uterine Cancer

Lanciano, R. M., Curran, W. J., Jr., Greven, K. M., Fanning, J., Stafford, P., Randall, M. E., & Hanks, G. E. (1990). Influence of grade, histologic subtype, and timing of radiotherapy on outcome among patients with stage II carcinoma of the endometrium. *Gynecologic Oncology, 39*(3), 368–373.

Leung, Y., & DePetrillo, A. D. (1993). Etiology, epidemiology, risk and prognostic factors, screening, and imaging of gynecologic cancers. *Current Opinion in Oncology, 5*(5), 869–876.

Photopulos, G. J. (1994). Surgicopathologic staging of endometrial adenocarcinoma. *Current Opinion in Obstetrics and Gynecology, 6*(1), 92–97.

Robert, M. E., & Fu, Y. S. (1990). Squamous cell carcinoma of the uterine cervix—a review with emphasis on prognostic factors and unusual variants. *Seminars in Diagnostic Pathology, 7*(3), 173–189.

Sarkaria, J. N., Petereit, D. G., Stitt, J. A., Hartman, T., Chappell, R., Thomadsen, B. R., Buchler, D. A., Fowler, J. F., & Kinsella, T. J. (1994). A comparison of the efficacy and complication rates of low dose-rate versus high dose-rate brachytherapy in the treatment of uterine cervical carcinoma. *International Journal of Radiation Oncology, Biology, Physics, 30*(1), 75–82.

Stock, R. J., Zaino, R., Bundy, B. N., Askin, F. B., Woodwardm, J., Fetter, B., Paulson, J. A., DiSaia, P. J., & Stehman, F. B. (1994). Evaluation and comparison of histopathologic grading systems of epithelial carcinoma of the uterine cervix: Gynecologic Oncology Group studies. *International Journal of Gynecological Pathology, 13*(2), 99–108.

Vaginal Cancer

Eddy, G. L., Marks, R. D., Jr., Miller, M. C., 3rd., & Underwood, P. B., Jr. (1991). Primary invasive vaginal carcinoma. *American Journal of Obstetrics and Gynecology, 165*(2), 292–296.

Franchi, M., & Donadello, N. (1994). Pelvic exenteration in gynecologic oncology. Review. *European Journal of Gynaecological Oncology, 15*(6), 469–474.

Manetta, A., Gutrecht, E. L., Berman, M. L., & DiSaia, P. J. (1990). Primary invasive carcinoma of the vagina. *Obstetrics and Gynecology, 76*(4), 639–642.

Vulvar Cancer

Hacker, N. F., & Van der Velden, J. (1993). Conservative management of early vulvar cancer. *Cancer, 71*(4, Suppl.), 1673–1677.

Hopkins, M. P., & Morley, G. W. (1992). Pelvic exenteration for the treatment of vulvar cancer. *Cancer, 70*(12), 2835–2838.

Penney, G. C., Kitchener, H. C., & Templeton, A. (1995). The management of carcinoma of the vulva: Current opinion and current practice among consultant gynaecologists in Scotland. *Health Bulletin, 53*(1), 47–54.

Petereit, D. G., Mehta, M. P., Buchler, D. A., & Kinsella, T. J. (1993). A retrospective review of nodal treatment for vulvar cancer. *American Journal of Clinical Oncology, 16*(1), 38–42.

Wilm's Tumor

Green, D. M., Beckwith, J. B., Weeks, D. A., Moksness, J., Breslow, N. E., & D'Angio, G. J. (1994). The relationship between microsubstaging variables, age at diagnosis, and tumor weight of children with stage I/favorable histology Wilms' tumor. A report from the National Wilms Tumor study. *Cancer, 74*(6), 1817–1820.

Marina, N. M., Wilimas, J. A., Meyer, W. H., Jones, D. P., Douglass, E. C., & Pratt, C. B. (1994). Refining therapeutic strategies for patients with resistant Wilms' tumor. *American Journal of Pediatric Hematology/Oncology, 16*(4), 296–300.

Ritchey, M. L., Green, D. M., Breslow, N. B., Moksness, J., & Norkool, P. (1995). Accuracy of current imaging modalities in the diagnosis of synchronous bilateral Wilms' tumor. A report from the National Wilms Tumor Study Group. *Cancer, 75*(2), 600–604.

Ritchey, M. L., Haase, G. M., & Shochat, S. (1993). Current management of Wilms' tumor. *Seminars in Surgical Oncology, 9*(6), 502–509.

Ritchey, M. L., Kelalis, P. P., Breslow, N., Etzioni, R., Evans, I., Haase, G. M., & D'Angio, G. J. (1992). Surgical complications after nephrectomy for Wilms' tumor. *Surgery, Gynecology and Obstetrics, 175*(6), 507–514.

Warrier, R. P., & Regueira, O. (1992). Wilms' tumor. *Pediatric Nephrology, 6*(4), 358–364.

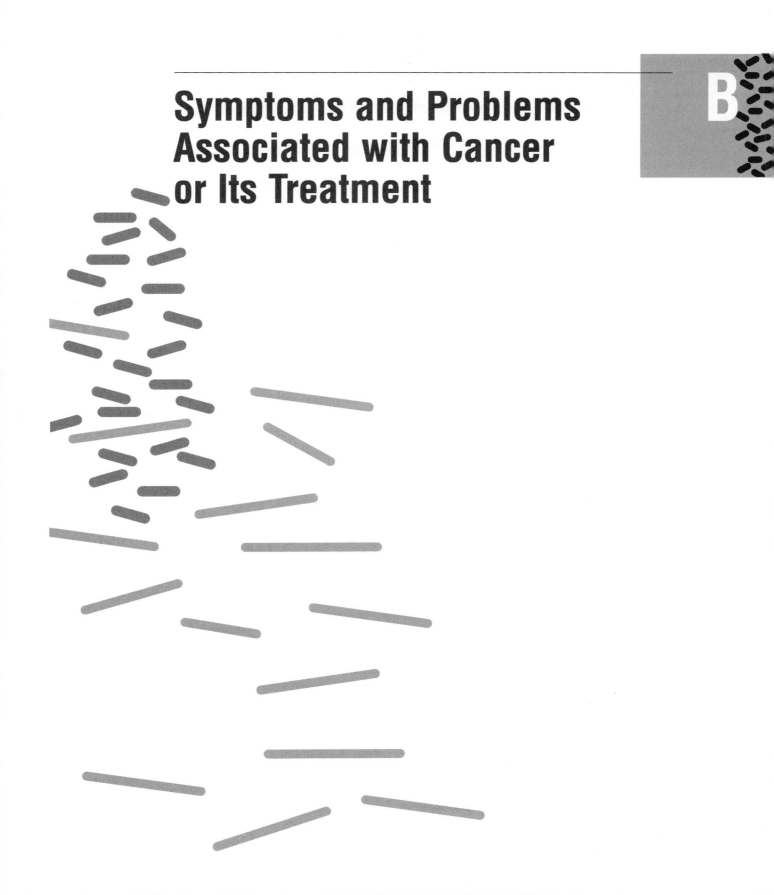

Symptoms and Problems Associated with Cancer or Its Treatment

B

Alopecia

Definition
- Temporary or permanent loss of hair that results from damage to and atrophy of the hair follicles incurred during cancer treatment

Etiology/Risk Factors
- Chemotherapy: cyclophosphamide, doxorubicin, vincristine, actinomycin D, bleomycin, cytosine arabinoside, daunorubicin, 5-FU, hydroxyurea, lomustine, methotrexate, mitomycin C, nitrogen mustard, semustine, vinblastine, vindesine, VM-26, VP-16-213, hexamethylmelamine
- Chronic stress
- Medical conditions: hyper-/hypothyroidism, hypoparathyroidism, Addison's disease, pernicious anemia, prolonged high fever
- Protein-calorie malnutrition
- Radiation therapy (1500–3000 cGy)

Assessment
- Examine other areas for hair loss: eyelashes, eyebrows, pubic hair, total body hair
- Examine the scalp

Diagnostic Tests
- None

Pharmacologic Management

- None

Nonpharmacologic Management

- Avoid use of hair dryers, curlers, curling irons, permanents, hair dyes
- Cut hair short
- Encourage discussion about feelings associated with hair loss
- Purchase wigs, hats, scarfs, turbans
- Use scalp hypothermia or tourniquet during chemotherapy
- Use a soft-bristled brush or a wide-toothed comb and minimize brushing and combing
- Wash scalp with a mild shampoo and minimize frequency of washes

Potential Problems
- Altered body image
- Depression
- Impaired sexual functioning

Anemia

Definition
• A reduction in the quantity and/or quality of RBCs to transport oxygen

Etiology/Risk Factors
• Blood loss
• Bone marrow failure from malignant disease (e.g., leukemia, lymphoma)
• Chemotherapy
• Infection
• Protein-calorie malnutrition
• Radiation therapy

Assessment
• Chest pain
• Difficulty concentrating
• Dizziness
• Dyspnea
• Fatigue
• Heart murmur
• Increased cold sensitivity
• Indigestion
• Irritability
• Pallor
• Syncope
• Tachycardia
• Weakness
• Widening pulse pressure

Diagnostic Tests
• CBC
• Coombs' Test
• RBC indices: MCV, MCH, MCHC
• Reticulocyte count
• Serum bilirubin
• Serum ferritin
• Serum iron level
• Total iron-binding capacity

Pharmacologic Management

• Iron supplements
• Oxygen, if necessary
• RBC transfusion

Nonpharmacologic Management

• Adequate nutrition
• Decrease activity
• Ensure warmth
• Promote rest

Potential Problems
• Fatigue
• Impaired mobility
• Myocardial infarction
• Potential for injury

Anorexia

Definition
- Loss of appetite or of the physiologic desire to eat

Etiology/Risk Factors
- Anxiety
- Chemotherapy
- Depression
- Fatigue
- Indirect effect of the cancer
- Nausea and vomiting
- Radiation therapy
- Stomatitis
- Surgery

Assessment
- Anthropometric measurements
- Bleeding or receding gums
- Brittle nails
- Flaky skin
- Height
- Poor dentition
- Thin, dull, dry hair
- Weight

Diagnostic Tests
- Serum albumin
- Skin tests for cell-mediated immunity
- Total lymphocyte count

Pharmacologic Management

- Administer vitamin supplements
- Hyperalimentation
- Nutritional supplements (e.g., Ensure, Carnation Instant Breakfast, Sustacal)

Nonpharmacologic Management

- Avoid fluid intake with meals
- Compile a food diary
- Consult with dietitian
- Encourage low-level exercise
- Encourage nutritional supplements
- Encourage "power-packed" (i.e., high-protein, high-calorie) foods
- Take brandy or sherry before meals
- Teach relaxation exercises to reduce anxiety

Potential Problems
- Anemia
- Dehydration
- Depression
- Fatigue
- Muscle wasting

Anxiety

Definition

• A sensation of apprehension of danger and dread accompanied by restlessness, tension, tachycardia, and dyspnea unattached to a clearly identifiable stimulus

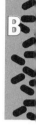

Etiology/Risk Factors

• Decision-making process
• Diagnosis of cancer
• Fear of the unknown
• Impending treatment
• Lack of understanding
• Uncertainty about prognosis

Assessment

• Anorexia and GI problems
• Constant demands
• Diaphoresis
• Elevated blood pressure
• Increased heart rate
• Increased questioning
• Increased respiratory rate
• Insomnia
• Restlessness
• Trembling

Diagnostic Tests

• None

Pharmacologic Management

• Antianxiety medications

Nonpharmacologic Management

• Encourage verbalization of feelings and concerns
• Establish a relaxed atmosphere
• Evaluate coping skills and teach new skills if necessary
• Evaluate need for psychiatric referral or psychological counseling
• Provide patient education
• Teach patient relaxation exercises

Potential Problems

• Anorexia
• Failure to adhere to the treatment regimen
• Panic attacks

Body Image Disturbance

Definition

- A state in which an individual perceives an alteration in the mental picture of his or her physical self

Etiology/Risk Factors

- Alopecia
- Changes induced by tumor growth (e.g., skin lesions, ascites)
- Cutaneous effects of chemotherapy or radiation therapy
- Disfiguring surgery

Assessment

- Anxiety
- Change in body structure
- Depression
- Expression of negative feelings about body
- Fear of rejection
- Ignores or fails to look at affected body part

Diagnostic Tests

- None

Pharmacologic Management

- Antidepressants
- Antianxiety medications

Nonpharmacologic Management

- Evaluate coping strategies and teach new skills if necessary
- Refer to a hair stylist or cosmetologist
- Reinforce any verbalizations of feelings about actual or perceived loss
- Reinforce attempts to attend to body part

Potential Problems

- Depression
- Panic attacks
- Suicidal ideation

Confusion

Definition

- A mental state in which reactions to environmental stimuli are inappropriate; a state in which a person is bewildered or perplexed or unable to orient her- or himself

Etiology/Risk Factors

- Alcohol
- Fluid and electrolyte imbalances (e.g., hyponatremia, hypercalcemia)
- Hypoxia
- Infectious processes
- Liver disease
- Medications: opioids, sedatives, barbiturates, anticholinergic drugs
- Neurodegenerative diseases
- Seizures
- Tumor growth

Assessment

- Anxiety
- Decreased attention span
- Dilated pupils
- Disorientation to time, place, person
- Inability to concentrate
- Insomnia
- Irritability
- Psychomotor restlessness
- Sweating
- Tachycardia
- Visual disturbances

Diagnostic Tests

- Arterial blood gases
- CT
- MRI
- Serum electrolyte levels

Pharmacologic Management

- Administer antipsychotics in small doses (e.g., haloperidol, 2 mg PO, at bedtime)
- Discontinue medications that may be contributing to the acute confusional state

Nonpharmacologic Management

- Obtain referral to a psychiatrist or psychologist if necessary
- Orient patient to time, place, and person on a regular basis
- Provide a pleasant, safe environment
- Put orientation devices (e.g., calendar, clock, family pictures) in patient's room

Potential Problems

- Potential for injury
- Impaired communication patterns

Constipation

Definition
• The passage, with discomfort or pain, of irregular, infrequent, hard feces

Etiology/Risk Factors
• Abdominal surgery
• Anxiety
• Chemotherapy: vincristine, vinblastine
• Decreased mobility
• Depression
• Hypercalcemia
• Inadequate dietary intake of fluid
• Inadequate dietary intake of roughage
• Medications: opioids, antidepressants, anticonvulsants, tranquilizers, muscle relaxants
• GI tract tumors

Assessment
• Abdominal distention or bloating
• Back pain
• Cramping abdominal pain or discomfort
• Decreased bowel sounds
• Decreased frequency of defecation
• Hard, formed, dry, or marble-sized stools
• Headache
• Interference with usual ADL
• Sensation of pressure in rectum
• Straining during defecation

Diagnostic Test
• Rectal examination

Pharmacologic Management
• Enemas
• Laxatives

Nonpharmacologic Management
• Avoidance of cheese products and refined grain products
• High-fiber diet
• Establish an exercise regimen with the patient
• Increase fluid intake (8–10-oz glasses per day)
• Obtain a dietary consult
• Teach patient to respond immediately to the urge to defecate

Potential Problems
• Decreased activity
• Fecal impaction
• Pain

Cystitis

Definition
• Inflammation of the urinary bladder

Etiology/Risk Factors
• Bacterial infections
• Chemotherapy: cyclophosphamide, ifosfamide
• Viral infections

Assessment
• Dysuria
• Frequency
• Hematuria
• Suprapubic discomfort
• Suprapubic tenderness
• Urgency

Diagnostic Tests
• Urinalysis
• Urine cultures

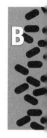

Pharmacologic Management

• Antimicrobial therapy: TMP-SMX (160/800 mg PO, q12h for 1–3 days); cephalexin (250–500 mg PO q6h for 1–3 days); ciprofloxacin (250–500 mg PO q12h for 1–3 days); or norfloxacine (400 mg PO q12h for 1–3 days)
• Mesna: IV dose equal to 20% of ifosfamide dose, at the same time as ifosfamide and 4 and 8 hours later

Nonpharmacologic Management

• Heating pad
• Relaxation exercises
• Sitz baths

Potential Problems
• Fatigue
• Insomnia
• Pain
• Sepsis

Depression: Reactive

Definition
- Depression in reaction to some outside adverse life situation, usually a crisis, loss of a person, or loss of an established role

Etiology/Risk Factors
- Diagnosis of cancer
- Disfiguring surgery
- Fatigue
- Pain
- Recurrence of cancer

Assessment
- Anger
- Anorexia
- Constipation
- Discouragement
- Fatigue
- Feelings of guilt
- Feelings of worthlessness
- Insomnia
- Irritability
- Lack of concentration
- Loss of interest and pleasure
- Mild sadness
- Weight loss
- Withdrawal from activities
- Worry

Diagnostic Tests
- None

Pharmacologic Management
- Analgesic medications (for pain management)
- Selective serotonin-reuptake inhibitors
- Tricyclic antidepressants

Nonpharmacologic Management
- Family counseling consultation
- Psychiatric consultation
- Social service referrals
- Structuring of patient's daily activities

Potential Problems
- Fatigue
- Ineffective family coping
- Self-care deficit
- Suicidal ideation

Diarrhea

Definition
• Frequent passage of stools of a soft or liquid consistency, with or without discomfort

Etiology/Risk Factors
• Anxiety
• Chemotherapy
• Dietary supplements with high osmolarity
• External radiation to the abdominal area
• Fecal impaction
• Infection
• Internal radiation to the uterus, cervix, or vagina
• Lactose intolerance
• Medications (e.g., antibiotics)
• Surgical intervention
• Tumors of the GI tract

Assessment
• Abdominal cramping
• Decreased skin turgor
• Flatus
• Increased bowel sounds
• Increase in the fluid content of the stool
• Increase in the number of bowel movements

Diagnostic Tests
• Intake and output
• Serum electrolytes
• Stool cultures
• Urine specific gravity

Pharmacologic Management

• Antianxiety medications
• Antidiarrhea medications
• Antispasmodic medications

Nonpharmacologic Management

• Eliminate foods and beverages that are irritating or stimulating to the GI tract
• Increase fluid intake to at least 3000 ml/day
• Initiate skin care measures to perirectal area, including sitz baths, A & D Ointment
• Obtain dietary consultation
• Prescribe a low-residue, high-protein and high-calorie diet

Potential Problems
• Dehydration
• Fatigue
• Malnutrition
• Pain
• Perirectal skin breakdown

Dysphagia

Definition
- Difficulty in swallowing

Etiology/Risk Factors
- Esophageal motility disorders
- Fibrosis
- Gastroesophageal reflux
- Infections
- Neuropathies
- Stomatitis/esophagitis
- Surgical resection
- Tumors of the head and neck

Assessment
- Choking when swallowing
- Coughing while eating
- Cough reflex
- Cranial nerve functioning
- Food sticking in pharynx or esophagus
- Gag reflex
- Oral cavity assessment
- Pain when swallowing
- Weakness of oral musculature

Diagnostic Test
- Swallowing assessment

Pharmacologic Management
- Analgesics, parenteral or topical
- Appropriate antibiotic therapy

Nonpharmacologic Management
- Begin oral exercises to strengthen lips, jaw, and tongue
- Obtain a consultation with a speech pathologist
- Offer small, frequent meals
- Place patient in a sitting position or high Fowler's, during and after meals
- Provide dietary supplements

Potential Problems
- Aspiration pneumonia
- Dehydration
- Fatigue
- Nutritional deficit
- Pain
- Respiratory arrest

Dsypnea

Definition

- Shortness of breath; a subjective difficulty or distress in breathing

Etiology/Risk Factors

- Anxiety
- Depression
- Fear
- Pain
- Pulmonary infections
- Pulmonary tumors or metastases

Assessment

- Depth of respiration
- Report of sensation of shortness of breath
- Respiratory rate
- Tachypnea
- Thoracic expansion

Diagnostic Tests

- Arterial blood gases
- Chest radiography
- Lung sounds
- Pulmonary function tests

Pharmacologic Management

- Antianxiety medications
- Bronchodilator therapy
- Opioid analgesics
- Oxygen therapy

Nonpharmacologic Management

- Teach energy conservation techniques
- Teach pursed-lips breathing and slow abdominal-diaphragmatic breathing
- Teach relaxation exercises
- Provide pillows and/or elevate head of bed

Potential Problems

- Decreased mobility
- Fatigue
- Insomnia
- Panic attack

Extravasation

Definition
- Inadvertent infiltration of IV fluids or medicines into the subcutaneous tissues surrounding an infusion site

Etiology/Risk Factors
- Lymphedema
- Poor venous access
- Superior vena cava syndrome
- Vesicant chemotherapy: nitrogen mustard, vincristine, vinblastine, actinomycin D, mithramycin, mitomycin C, doxorubicin, daunomycin, DTIC, streptozotocin

Assessment
- Burning
- Erythema
- Fibrosis of blood vessel
- Lack of blood return
- Pain
- Skin browning
- Swelling
- Ulceration

Diagnostic Tests
- None

Pharmacologic Management

- Hyaluronidase: subcutaneous injection around insertion site
- Hydrocortisone sodium succinate: SC or intradermal injection around injection site
- Sodium bicarbonate (8.2%): SC administration or IV administration through the needle or catheter
- Sodium thiosulfate (10%) instilled into the vein and tissue area
- Topical corticosteroid cream

Non-pharmacologic Management

- Apply cold to area (heat, if a vinca alkaloid)
- Consider placement of a venous access device
- Elevate the extremity

Potential Problems
- Impaired functioning of the extremity
- Infection
- Pain

Fatigue: Acute

Definition
- A feeling of weariness, weakness, depletion, and exhaustion or an inability to mobilize energy to carry on that is associated with a desire for sleep and rest; lasting less than 1 month

Etiology/Risk Factors
- Anemia
- Anxiety
- Chemotherapy
- Immobility
- Insomnia
- Pain
- Protein-calorie malnutrition
- Radiation therapy
- Sensory deprivation

Assessment
- Agitation
- Anorexia
- Apathy
- Decreased ability to make decisions
- Feelings of hopelessness and helplessness
- Impaired concentration and memory
- Insomnia
- Irritability
- Pattern of fatigue
- Tearfulness
- Usual rest and sleep pattern
- Withdrawal

Diagnostic Test
- CBC

Pharmacologic Management

- Transfusion of packed RBCs, if necessary

Nonpharmacologic Management

- Implement an exercise program that is individualized to the patient's physical and psychosocial status
- Obtain physical and occupational therapy referrals
- Obtain support services
- Teach patient to pace activities

Potential Problems
- Depression
- Nutritional deficit
- Suicidal ideation

Fatigue: Chronic

Definition
- A feeling of weariness, weakness, depletion, and exhaustion or an inability to mobilize energy to carry on that is associated with a desire for sleep and rest; persisting longer than 1 month

Etiology/Risk Factors
- Anemia
- Anxiety
- Chemotherapy
- Immobility
- Insomnia
- Pain
- Protein-calorie malnutrition
- Radiation therapy
- Sensory deprivation

Assessment
- Agitation
- Anorexia
- Apathy
- Decreased ability to make decisions
- Feelings of hopelessness and helplessness
- Impaired concentration and memory
- Insomnia
- Irritability
- Pattern of fatigue
- Tearfulness
- Usual rest and sleep pattern
- Withdrawal

Diagnostic Test
- CBC

Pharmacologic Management

- Transfusion of packed RBCs, if necessary

Nonpharmacologic Management

- Implement an exercise program that is individualized to the patient's physical and psychosocial status
- Obtain physical and occupational therapy referrals
- Obtain support services
- Teach patient to pace activities
- Use distraction, support groups, and/or cognitive-behavioral approaches to reduce fatigue

Potential Problems
- Depression
- Nutritional deficit
- Suicidal ideation

Flulike Syndrome

Definition
- Constitutional effects often described as an influenza-like syndrome that occurs in patients receiving certain biologic and chemotherapeutic agents

Etiology/Risk Factors
- GM-CSF
- High-dose dacarbazine
- IL-1
- IL-2
- IFN-α
- Intravesical BCG
- TNF

Assessment
- Arthralgias
- Chills
- Diarrhea
- Dizziness
- Fever
- Headache
- Light-headedness
- Malaise
- Myalgias
- Nasal congestion
- Nausea
- Vomiting

Diagnostic Tests
- None

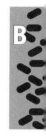

Pharmacologic Management
- Analgesics
- Antipyretics
- Pretreatment with nonsteroidal antiinflammatory drugs

Nonpharmacologic Management
- Adequate hydration
- Adequate rest
- Frequent linen changes
- Tepid sponge baths

Potential Problems
- Dehydration
- Fatigue
- Pain

Hypervolemia

Definition
- A state in which an individual experiences an increase in fluid volume related to increased fluid intake or decreased loss of fluid, volume shifts within body fluid compartments, or a combination thereof

Etiology/Risk Factors
- Congestive heart failure
- Hyperaldosteronism
- Increased intake of fluids
- Increased intake of sodium
- Renal insufficiency
- Severe stress
- Steroid therapy

Assessment
- Abnormal breath sounds
- Anorexia
- Anxiety
- Bounding pulses
- Change in blood pressure
- Changes in level of consciousness
- Dyspnea
- Edema
- Increased CVP
- Jugular venous distention
- Restlessness
- S_3 gallop
- Tachycardia
- Tachypnea
- Weight gain

Diagnostic Tests
- Arterial blood gases
- BUN
- Hematocrit
- Pulmonary artery catheterization
- Serum electrolytes
- Urine osmolality
- Urine specific gravity

Pharmacologic Management
- Diuretic therapy

Nonpharmacologic Management
- Daily weight
- Fluid restriction
- Maintain mobility

Potential Problems
- Pulmonary edema
- Skin breakdown

Hypovolemia

Definition

- A state of decreased circulating fluid volume related to decreased intake, or increased loss, of fluid, volume shifts within body fluid compartments, or a combination thereof

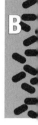

Etiology/Risk Factors

- Anorexia
- Ascites
- Capillary leak syndrome
- Diaphoresis
- Diarrhea
- Draining wounds
- Fistulas
- Hemorrhage
- Intestinal obstruction
- Nasogastric drainage
- Nausea and vomiting
- Sepsis
- Surgery

Assessment

- Change in mental status
- Decreased skin turgor
- Dizziness
- Dry mucous membranes
- Dry skin
- Hypotension
- Lethargy
- Postural hypotension
- Tachycardia
- Tachypnea
- Thirst
- Weakness

Diagnostic Tests

- BUN
- Hematocrit
- Serum osmolality
- Serum sodium
- Urine osmolality
- Urine specific gravity

Pharmacologic Management

- Blood component therapy
- IV fluids
- Volume expanders (e.g., albumin, dextran)

Nonpharmacologic Management

- Intake and output measurement
- Mouth care
- Skin care

Potential Problems

- Injury
- Renal failure
- Self-care deficit

Hypoxemia

Definition
• Suboptimal oxygenation of the blood

Etiology/Risk Factors
• Bronchitis
• Cardiac tamponade
• Emphysema
• Pneumonia
• Pulmonary fibrosis
• Pulmonary tumor or metastasis
• Septic shock
• Superior vena cava syndrome

Assessment
• Agitation
• Arrhythmias
• Bradycardia
• Confusion
• Cyanosis
• Depression
• Dyspnea
• Fatigue
• Restlessness
• Somnolence
• Tachycardia
• Tachypnea

Diagnostic Tests
• Arterial blood gases
• Hematocrit
• Pulmonary function tests

Pharmacologic Management
• Appropriate therapy for the underlying cause
• Bronchodilator therapy
• Oxygen therapy

Nonpharmacologic Management
• Chest physical therapy
• Encourage coughing and deep breathing
• Endotracheal suctioning
• High Fowler's position
• Incentive spirometer
• Pulmonary hygiene measures

Potential Problems
• Anxiety
• Fatigue
• Pain
• Potential for injury
• Self-care deficit

Impotence

Definition
• Inability to achieve penile erection

Etiology/Risk Factors
• Abdominoperineal resection
• Cancer treatment
• Surviving cancer and cancer treatment

Assessment
• History related to impotence
  • Course of events
  • Onset of problem
  • Patient's perception of problem
• Reproductive/contraceptive history
• Sexual history

Diagnostic Tests
• None

Pharmacologic Management

• None

Nonpharmacologic Management

• Encourage alternate forms of sexual activity: fondling, kissing, hugging
• Penile prosthesis
• Psychological counseling
• Treat other potential problems

Potential Problems
• Anxiety
• Depression
• Fatigue
• Stress

Infection: Eyes

Definiton
- A state in which the eyes are invaded by pathogenic microbes (i.e., bacteria, viruses, protozoa, fungi, yeasts) that have the ability to multiply under favorable conditions and cause cellular injury or destruction

Etiology/Risk Factors
- AIDS
- Antibiotic therapy
- BMT
- Chronic stress
- Leukemia
- Leukopenia
- Lymphoma
- Malnutrition
- Myeloma
- Steroids
- Surgery

Assessment
- Clarity
- Drainage
- Presence of eyelashes
- Redness

Diagnostic Tests
- Culture and sensitivity

Pharmacologic Management
- Antimicrobial therapy based on culture and sensitivity reports

Nonpharmacologic Management
- Artificial lubricants as needed
- Strict hand washing

Potential Problems
- Blindness
- Pain
- Injury
- Pruritus

Infection: Genitourinary Tract

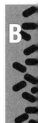

Definition
- A state in which the GU tract is invaded by pathogenic microbes (i.e., bacteria, viruses, protozoa, fungi, yeasts) that have the ability to multiply under favorable conditions and cause cellular injury or destruction

Etiology/Risk Factors
- AIDS
- Antibiotic therapy
- BMT
- Chronic stress
- Leukemia
- Leukopenia
- Lymphoma
- Malnutrition
- Myeloma
- Steroids
- Surgery

Assessment
- Dysuria
- Flank pain
- Frequency
- Urgency
- Urine: color, clarity, odor
- Voiding patterns

Diagnostic Tests
- CBC
- Residual urine volumes
- Urinalysis
- Urine culture and sensitivity
- VDRL and gonococcal smears
- WBC with differential

Pharmacologic Management
- Antimicrobial therapy based on culture and sensitivity reports
- Bladder analgesics: phenazopyridine and flavoxate

Nonpharmacologic Management
- Alkalinization of urine (with cranberry juice)
- Avoid indwelling catheter
- Ensure fluid intake of 3000 ml per day, unless contraindicated
- Perineal hygiene measures

Potential Problems
- Dehydration
- Pain
- Renal insufficiency
- Sepsis

Infection: Mucous Membranes

Definition
- A state in which the mucous membranes are invaded by pathogenic microbes (i.e., bacteria, viruses, protozoa, fungi, yeasts) that have the ability to multiply under favorable conditions and cause cellular injury or destruction

Etiology/Risk Factors
- AIDS
- Antibiotic therapy
- BMT
- Chronic Stress
- Leukemia
- Leukopenia
- Lymphoma
- Malnutrition
- Myeloma
- Steroids
- Surgery

Assessment
- Characteristics
  - Color
  - Edema
  - Lesions
  - Moisture
- Locations
  - Oral cavity
  - Rectum
  - Vagina

Diagnostic Tests
- CBC
- Culture and sensitivity
- WBC with differential

Pharmacologic Management
- Appropriate antimicrobial therapy based on culture and sensitivity reports
- (See Mucositis: Chemotherapy-Induced)

Nonpharmacologic Management
- Avoid enemas, rectal medications, rectal temperatures, digital rectal examinations
- Oral care regimen
- Wound irrigations

Potential Problems
- Pain
- Skin breakdown

Infection: Respiratory Tract

Definition

- A state in which the respiratory tract is invaded by pathogenic microbes (i.e., bacteria, viruses, protozoa, fungi, yeasts) that have the ability to multiply under favorable conditions and cause cellular injury or destruction

Etiology/Risk Factors

- AIDS
- Antibiotic therapy
- BMT
- Chronic stress
- Leukemia
- Leukopenia
- Lymphoma
- Malnutrition
- Myeloma
- Steroids
- Surgery

Assessment

- Cough
- Dyspnea
- Pleuritic pain
- Respiratory assessment
- Sputum: color, amount
- Tachycardia
- Tachypenia

Diagnostic Tests

- Arterial blood gases
- Chest radiography
- Pulmonary function tests
- Sputum culture and sensitivity
- Tuberculosis skin test

Pharmacologic Management

- Antimicrobial therapy based on culture and sensitivity reports
- Humidification and nebulizing mist treatments
- Oxygen therapy

Nonpharmacologic Management

- Incentive spirometry
- Nasopharyngeal suctioning
- Pulmonary hygiene
- Reduce environmental contaminants

Potential Problems

- Anxiety
- Dyspnea
- Fatigue
- Impaired gas exchange
- Impaired mobility
- Pain

Infection: Skin

Definition
- A state in which the skin is invaded by pathogenic microbes (i.e., bacteria, viruses, protozoa, fungi, yeasts) that have the ability to multiply under favorable conditions and cause cellular injury or destruction

Etiology/Risk Factors
- AIDS
- Antibiotic therapy
- BMT
- Chronic stress
- Leukemia
- Leukopenia
- Lymphoma
- Malnutrition
- Myeloma
- Steroids
- Surgery

Assessment
- Skin assessment: characteristics
  - Color
  - Edema
  - Lesions, wounds, fissures
  - Moisture
- Skin assessment: locations
  - Bony prominences
  - IV or puncture sites
  - Skinfolds
  - Venous access devices
- Wound assessment
  - Drainage
  - Inflammation
  - Odor
  - Tenderness

Diagnostic Tests
- CBC
- Skin/wound cultures
- WBC with differential

Pharmacologic Management

- Appropriate antimicrobial therapy based on culture and sensitivity reports

Nonpharmacologic Management

- Meticulous skin care
- Meticulous technique with venipunctures and other invasive procedures
- Prevent skin abrasions
- Use only electric razor or depilatory

Potential Problems
- Pain
- Pressure ulcers
- Tissue necrosis
- Ulcerated wounds

Infection: Systemic

Definition
- A state in which the body is invaded by pathogenic microbes (i.e., bacteria, viruses, protozoa, fungi, yeasts) that have the ability to multiply under favorable conditions and cause cellular injury or destruction

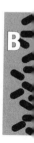

Etiology/Risk Factors
- AIDS
- Antibiotic therapy
- BMT
- Chronic stress
- Leukemia
- Leukopenia
- Lymphoma
- Malnutrition
- Myeloma
- Steroids
- Surgery

Assessment
- CNS assessment
- Cardiovascular assessment
- Examine all secretions
- Fluid balance evaluation
- Inspect all body sites
- Respiratory assessment
- Temperature

Diagnostic Tests
- Anergy skin testing
- Appropriate cultures (blood, urine, wound, stool, sputum)
- CBC
- WBC with differential

Pharmacologic Management
- Colony-stimulating factors (to promote hematopoiesis)
- Antimicrobial therapy based on culture and sensitivity reports

Nonpharmacologic Management
- Adequate hydration
- Fever management
- High-protein, high-calorie diet
- Protective isolation
- Strict hand washing

Potential Problems
- Dehydration
- Fatigue
- Nutritional deficit
- Pain

Infertility: Female

Definition
- Altered ovarian function that prevents ovulation and subsequent successful fertilization and implantation of the products of conception

Etiology/Risk Factors
- Bilateral oophorectomy
- Chemotherapy: especially the alkylating agents (chlorambucil, cyclophosphamide), doxorubicin, cytarabine, procarbazine, vinblastine, busulfan
- Hysterectomy
- Radiation to the lower abdomen, pelvis, gonads

Assessment
- Menstrual history
- Reproductive/contraceptive history
- Sexual history
- Symptoms of estrogen deficiency: hot flashes, vaginal dryness, dyspareunia

Diagnostic Tests
- Serum LH
- Serum FSH

Pharmacologic Management
- Exogenous estrogens

Nonpharmacologic Management
- Family counseling
- Oophoropexy (surgical displacement of the ovaries) outside the radiation treatment field during pelvic irradiation
- Psychological support
- Reproductive counseling
- Shielding the ovaries during radiation therapy

Potential Problems
- Altered body image
- Anxiety
- Depression

Infertility: Male

Definition
- Alterations in sperm number, morphology, or motility that preclude successful fertilization of an ovum during copulation

Etiology/Risk Factors
- Bilateral orchiectomy
- Chemotherapy, especially with the alkylating agents (chlorambucil, cyclophosphamide), doxorubicin, cytarabine, procarbazine, vinblastine, busulfan, antiestrogen therapy
- Radiation to the lower abdomen, pelvis, gonads

Assessment
- Reproductive/contraceptive history
- Sexual history

Diagnostic Tests
- Serum FSH
- Serum testosterone
- Sperm count
- Testicular volume

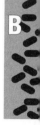

Pharmacologic Management
- Hypothalamic-releasing hormones (investigational)

Nonpharmacologic Management
- Artificial insemination
- Family counseling
- Psychological support
- Reproductive counseling
- Shielding of testes during radiation therapy
- Sperm banking

Potential Problems
- Altered body image
- Anxiety
- Depression
- Impaired sexual functioning

Insomnia

Definition
- Inability to sleep. Insomnia can be classified as one of three types: initial (difficulty in falling asleep), intermittent (inability to stay asleep), and terminal (early morning awakening)

Etiology/Risk Factors
- Biotherapy
- Cancer diagnosis
- Chemotherapy
- Radiation therapy
- Surgery
- Symptoms associated with the disease or treatment

Assessment
- Anxiety
- Depression
- Irritability
- Loss of train of thought
- Mental confusion
- Number and timing of naps
- Usual sleep pattern
  - Time of retirement
  - Time needed to fall asleep
  - Number of awakenings
  - Intrusive thoughts
  - Total sleep time
  - Time of morning awakening

Diagnostic Tests
- None

Pharmacologic Management

- Use appropriate medications to provide symptomatic relief and enhance sleep
  - Psychotropic drugs
  - Sedatives
  - Hypnotics
  - Antianxiety medications
  - Tricyclic antidepressants
  - Antihistamines

Nonpharmacologic Management

- Adhere to patient's usual sleep-wake routines
- Administer back rub
- Avoid excessive stimulation at bedtime
- Decrease fluid intake at bedtime to avoid nocturia
- Decrease noise and sensory stimulation at bedtime
- Develop an appropriate exercise regimen
- Modify diet to avoid heavy meals and caffeine at bedtime
- Provide usual sleep environment

Potential Problems
- Depression
- Fatigue
- Cognitive impairment
- Confusion

Lymphedema

Definition

- Swelling in subcutaneous tissues as a result of obstruction of lymphatic vessels or lymph nodes and the accumulation of large amounts of lymph in the affected region

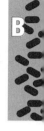

Etiology/Risk Factors

- Anemia
- Hypoalbuminemia
- Immobility
- Increasing tumor burden pressing or blocking the lymphatic system
- Infection
- Liver metastases
- Obesity
- Radiation therapy to the lymphatics
- Surgical resection of the lymphatics

Assessment

- Brown, woody skin texture
- Change in color of extremity
- Change in extremity sensation
- Change in fit of clothing/jewelry
- Change in size of extremity
- Coolness of skin
- Decreased ROM
- Discomfort of extremity
- Pitting edema
- Translucent skin

Diagnostic Tests

- None

Pharmacologic Management

- Diuretic therapy
- Parenteral albumin, as necessary

Nonpharmacologic Management

- Consult with physical therapist
- Elevate extremity
- ROM exercises
- Skin care
- Use assistive devices (e.g., intermittent pressure pump)
- Use elastic support devices

Potential Problems

- Decreased mobility
- Pain
- Potential for injury
- Self-care deficit
- Skin breakdown

Mucositis: Chemotherapy-Induced

Definition
- Inflammatory responses of the oral mucosa and intraoral soft tissue structures to the cytotoxic effects of chemotherapy

Etiology/Risk Factors
- BMT
- Chemotherapeutic drugs
  - Bleomycin
  - Dactinomycin
  - Daunorubicin
  - Doxorubicin
  - 5-Fluorouracil
  - Methotrexate
  - Vinblastine
- Dehydration
- Exposure to tobacco or alcohol
- Immunosuppression
- Malnutrition
- Poor oral hygiene

Assessment
- Examination of oral cavity
  - Clean teeth
  - Moist, soft lips
  - Pink and firm gingiva
  - Pink, moist mucosa and tongue
  - Saliva present
- Signs of oral infection
  - Candidiasis: cottage cheese–like white patches
  - Gram-negative organisms: creamy white, raised, shiny, nonpurulent, painful erosions on a reddened base
  - Gram-positive organisms: dry, raised, wartlike, yellowish brown, round placques
  - Herpes simplex: painful, itchy vesicles

Diagnostic Test
- KOH stain

Pharmacologic Management
- Appropriate antibiotic or antiviral therapy
- Artificial saliva
- Mild analgesics
  - Lidocaine HCl, diphenhydramine (12.5 mg/ml), and Maalox (equal parts)
  - Lidocaine HCl, 2 or 5% orally
- Oral care solution
  - Sodium bicarbonate solution (e.g., 1 tsp in 8 oz of water)
  - Sodium chloride (½ tsp) and sodium bicarbonate (1 tsp) solution (mix in 1 L water)
- Systemic analgesics

Nonpharmacologic Management
- Avoid foods that are thermally, chemically, or mechanically irritating
- Avoid use of alcohol or tobacco
- Dental consult
- High-protein diet
- Soft toothbrush

Potential Problems
- Dehydration
- Nutritious deficit
- Pain
- Sepsis

Mucositis: Radiation Therapy–Induced

Definition
- Inflammatory responses of the oral mucosa and intraoral soft tissue structures to the cytotoxic effects of radiation therapy

Etiology/Risk Factors
- Concomitant administration of chemotherapy
- Dehydration
- Exposure to tobacco or alcohol
- Immunosuppression
- Malnutrition
- Poor oral hygiene
- Radiation therapy to the head and neck region

Assessment
- Examination of oral cavity
  - Clean teeth
  - Moist, soft lips
  - Pink and firm gingiva
  - Pink, moist mucosa and tongue
  - Saliva present
- Signs of oral infection
  - Candidiasis: cottage cheese-like white patches
  - Gram-negative: creamy white, raised, shiny, nonpurulent, painful erosions on a reddened base
  - Gram-positive: dry, raised, wartlike, yellowish brown, round placques
  - Herpes simplex: painful, itchy vesicles

Diagnostic Test
- KOH stain

Pharmacologic Management
- Appropriate antibiotic or antiviral therapy
- Artificial saliva
- Mild analgesics
  - Lidocaine HCl, diphenhydramine (12.5 mg/ml), and Maalox (equal parts)
  - Lidocaine HCl 2 or 5% orally
- Oral care solution
  - Sodium bicarbonate solution (e.g., 1 tsp in 8 oz of water)
  - Sodium chloride (½ tsp) and sodium bicarbonate (1 tsp) solution (mix in 1 L water)
- Systemic analgesics

Nonpharmacologic Management
- Avoid foods that are thermally, chemically, or mechanically irritating
- Avoid use of alcohol or tobacco
- Dental consult
- High-protein diet
- Soft toothbrush

Potential Problems
- Dehydration
- Nutritional deficit
- Pain
- Sepsis

Nausea and Vomiting: Acute

Definition

• *Nausea,* an awareness of the urge to vomit, is associated with a loss of gastric tone and motility and with reflux of the duodenal contents into the stomach. *Vomiting* is coordinated expulsion of gastric contents

Etiology/Risk Factors

• Biologic response modifiers
• Chemotherapy
• Gastric outlet obstruction
• Gastrointestinal cancers
• Hepatic metastasis
• Hypercalcemia
• Increased intracranial pressure
• Opioid analgesics
• Radiation therapy
• Uremia

Assessment

• Decreased skin turgor
• Dietary history
• Flushing
• Pallor
• Salivation
• Self-report of severity of nausea
• Sweating
• Tachycardia/bradycardia
• Vomiting: amount, frequency, color, odor
• Weight

Diagnostic Tests

• Anthropomorphic measurements
• BUN
• Diagnostic radiography
• Serum electrolytes

Pharmacologic Management

• Benzamides: metoclopramide (2 mg/kg q2h $\times$ 5 doses; 3 mg/kg q2h $\times$ 2 doses; 3 mg/kg load, then 0.5 mg/kg/h for 12 h; 0.5–3 mg/kg q2–6h)
• Butyrophenones: haloperidol (1–3 mg q2–8h); droperidol (10 mg, then 4 mg q2h $\times$ 4 doses)
• Cannabinoids: dronabinol (5–10 mg/m^2 q3–4h)
• Corticosteroids: dexamethasone (10–20 mg q6–12h); methylprednisolone (125–500 mg q6h)
• Phenothiazines: prochlorperazine (5–10 mg q4–6h); thiethylperazine (25 mg q6–8h); perphenazine (4–6 mg q6h)
• Serotonin antagonists: ondansetron (0.15 mg/kg q4h $\times$ 3 doses; 0.3 mg/kg pre- and 3.5 hours postchemotherapy; 8 mg IV load, then 1 mg/h for 24 hours; 32 mg for 1 dose prechemotherapy 8 mg q8h for 2–3 days); granisetron (10 μg over 5 minutes)

Nonpharmacologic Management

• Behavior modification
• Diversional activity
• Hypnosis
• Meditation
• Quiet, restful environment
• Relaxation techniques
• Small, frequent, nutritious meals

Potential Complications

• Dehydration
• Esophageal tear
• Protein-calorie malnutrition

Nausea and Vomiting: Anticipatory

Definition
• The occurrence of nausea and vomiting prior to cancer treatment

Etiology/Risk Factors
• Negative experiences or feelings toward chemotherapy
• Sensations of tastes and odors
• Severe nausea and vomiting that was inadequately controlled
• Younger age

Assessment
• Level of anxiety
• Nutritional intake
• Pattern of nausea and vomiting
• Previous experiences associated with cancer treatment
• Responses to environmental stimuli
• Responses to food and fluids

Diagnostic Tests
• None

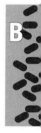

Pharmacologic Management

• Institute effective antiemetic regimen

Nonpharmacologic Management

• Behavior modification
• Biofeedback
• Desensitization
• Dietary modifications
• Diversional therapy
• Guided imagery
• Hypnosis
• Meditation
• Mouth care regimen
• Relaxation therapy

Potential Problems
• Anxiety
• Dehydration
• Failure to adhere to treatment schedule
• Fatigue
• Nutritional deficit

Oral Candidiasis

Definition

- Superficial fungal infection of the oral mucosa

Etiology/Risk Factors

- Dehydration
- Exposure to tobacco and alcohol
- External radiation therapy to the head and neck
- Immunosuppression
- Poor oral hygiene
- Protein-calorie malnutrition

Assessment

- Burning sensation
- Cottage cheese–like white patches
- Metallic taste
- Reddened, ulcerated skin surface below white patches

Diagnostic Test

- KOH smear

Pharmacologic Management

- Nystatin: 1.5 million units PO, t.i.d.
- Fluconazole: 50 mg/day PO
- Ketoconazole: 200 mg/day PO

Nonpharmacologic Management

- Avoid foods that are thermally, chemically, or physically irritating
- Avoid tobacco and alcohol
- Dental consult
- Oral hygiene protocol
- Soft toothbrush

Potential Problems

- Dehydration
- Infection (systemic)
- Nutritional deficit
- Pain

Oral Herpes Simplex

Definition
· Superficial viral infection of the oral mucosa

Etiology/Risk Factors
· Dehydration
· Exposure to tobacco and alcohol
· External radiation therapy to the head and neck
· Immunosuppression
· Poor oral hygiene
· Protein-calorie malnutrition

Assessment
· Encrusted, dry exudate
· Painful, itching vesicles
· Stinging
· First vesicles on lips

Diagnostic Tests
· Tzanck smear
· Viral culture

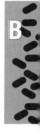

Pharmacologic Management

· Acyclovir: 200 mg PO, q4h, five times a day for 10–14 days

Nonpharmacologic Management

· Avoid foods that are thermally, chemically, or physically irritating
· Avoid tobacco and alcohol
· Dental consult
· Oral hygiene protocol
· Soft toothbrush

Potential Problems
· Dehydration
· Infection (systemic)
· Nutritional deficit
· Pain

Pain: Acute Postoperative

Definition
- An unpleasant sensory and emotional experience associated with actual tissue damage resulting from some type of surgical procedure

Etiology/Risk Factor
- Surgery

Assessment
- Pain history
  - Aggravating and relieving factors
  - Description
  - Intensity/severity
  - Location and radiation
  - Previous treatment modalities and efficacy
- Behavioral/Physiologic Manifestations
  - Agitation
  - Blood pressure changes
  - Crying
  - Guarding behavior
  - Heart rate changes
  - Immobility
  - Respiratory rate changes
  - Restlessness
  - Vocalizations

Diagnostic Tests
- None

Pharmacologic Management

- Nonopioid analgesics
- Opioid analgesics
  - IV (PCA)
  - Oral
  - Spinal

Nonpharmacologic Management

- Distraction
- Preoperative patient education
- Relaxation therapy
- TENS

Potential Problems
- Anxiety
- Immobility
- Insomnia
- Pneumonia

Pain: Acute, Procedure-Related

Definition
- An unpleasant sensory and emotional experience associated wtih actual tissue damage resulting from some type of invasive procedure

Etiology/Risk Factors
- Diagnostic procedures
- Therapeutic procedures

Assessment
- Knowledge of the procedure
- Level of anxiety
- Previous experience with the procedure

Diagnostic Tests
- None

Pharmacologic Management

- Benzodiazepines: provide anxiolysis, skeletal muscle relaxation, and, at higher doses, amnesia (e.g., midazolam, 0.5-mg increments, IV)
- Local anesthetics: local infiltration or topical application (e.g., eutectic mixture of local anesthetics [EMLA])
- Opioids: often administered intravenously (e.g., morphine 2 to 4 mg q5min; fentanyl 25-μg increments, very slowly)
- Treat procedure-related pain prophylactically

Nonpharmacologic Management

- Counterstimulation
- Distraction
- Hypnosis
- Relaxation

Potential Problems
- Anxiety
- Failure to adhere to the diagnostic or therapeutic regimen
- Fear

Pain: Bone Metastasis

Definition
• Pain caused by tumor infiltration of bone

Etiology/Risk Factors
• Breast
• Kidney
• Lung
• Multiple myeloma
• Prostate
• Thyroid

Assessment
• Muscle spasms
• Pain
  • Constant
  • Worsens with movement
  • Worsens at night
  • Worsens with weight bearing

Diagnostic Tests
• Bone scan
• MRI
• Skeletal radiography

Pharmacologic Management

• Nonsteroidal antiinflammatory drugs
• Opioid analgesics
• Steroids

Nonpharmacologic Management

• Acupuncture
• Distraction
• Hypnosis
• Radiation therapy: desired dose of radiation should be administered in the fewest fractions possible, to promote patient comfort during and after treatment
• Radiopharmaceuticals
  • Iodine 131 for bony metastases from thyroid cancer
  • Phosphorus 32 for bony metastases from breast and prostate cancer
  • Strontium 89
• Relaxation and imagery
• Use of heat or cold

Potential Problems
• Depression
• Fatigue
• Impaired mobility
• Pathologic fractures
• Self-care deficit
• Spinal cord compression

Pain: Neuropathic

Definition
- Pain initiated or caused by a primary lesion or dysfunction in the nervous system

Etiology/Risk Factors
- Base of skull metastases
- Chemotherapy: vincristine, cisplatin, taxol
- Leptomeningeal disease
- Postherpetic neuralgia
- Radiation-induced damage to peripheral nerves
- Surgery
  - Limb amputation
  - Mastectomy
  - Nephrectomy
  - Radical head and neck
  - Thoracotomy

Assessment
- Allodynia
- Atrophy
- Hair loss
- Hyperalgesia
- Loss of reflexes
- Pain
  - Aching
  - Burning
  - Dysesthesias
  - Sharp, lancinating
- Sensory loss
- Smooth, fine skin

Diagnostic Tests
- EMG
- Somatosensory testing

Pharmacologic Management

- Anticonvulsants (for stabbing, shocklike component)
  - Carbamazepine, 200–1600 mg/day PO
  - Phenytoin, 300–500 mg/day PO
- Antidepressants
  - Amitriptyline, 25–150 mg/day PO
  - Doxepin, 25–150 mg/day PO
  - Imipramine, 20–100 mg/day PO
  - Trazadone, 75–225 mg/day PO
- Local anesthesias
  - Lidocaine, 5 mg/kg, IV
  - Mexiletine, 450–600 mg/day PO
  - Tocainide, 20 mg/kg/day PO

Nonpharmacologic Management

- Acupuncture
- Distraction
- Hypnosis
- Relaxation and imagery
- TENS

Potential Problems
- Depression
- Fatigue
- Impaired mobility
- Potential for injury
- Self-care deficit

Pain: Visceral

Definition
• Pain that originates from injury to sympathetically innervated organs

Etiology/Risk Factors
• Acute ischemia
• Chemical irritation
• Distension of the capsule of a solid viscus
• Gastrointestinal malignancies
• Hepatic metastases
• Infectious peritonitis
• Inflammation of the parietal peritoneum
• Invasion or compression of a nerve root
• Obstruction of a hollow viscus
• Omental metastasis
• Thrombosis and engorgement of splenic and renal veins

Assessment
• BP changes
• Diaphoresis
• Distention
• Feeling of fullness
• Heart rate changes
• Nausea and vomiting
• Pain
  • Aching
  • Deep
  • Dull
  • Paroxysmal, colicky
  • Pressurelike
  • Squeezing
  • Vague distribution
  • Vague quality

Diagnostic Tests
• Abdominal CT
• Abdominal radiography

Pharmacologic Management

• Antiemetic therapy
• Laxatives (if appropriate)
• Nonopioid analgesics
• Opioid analgesics

Nonpharmacologic Management

• Acupuncture
• Chemotherapy
• Distraction
• Hypnosis
• Mechanical decompression of an obstruction
• Nerve blocks
• Radiation therapy
• Relaxation and imagery
• Surgery

Potential Problems
• Depression
• Dehydration
• Fatigue
• Nutritional deficit
• Self-care deficit

Peripheral Neuropathy

Definition
- Constant or intermittent burning, aching, or lancinating limb pain due to generalized or focal disease of peripheral nerves

Etiology/Risk Factors
- Cisplatin
- Compression of a peripheral nerve
- Myeloma
- Radiation-induced damage to peripheral nerves
- Taxol
- Tumor infiltration of a peripheral nerve
- Vincristine

Assessment
- Allodynia
- Atrophy
- Hair loss
- Hyperalgesia
- Pain
  - Aching
  - Burning
  - Distal pain
  - Dysesthesias
  - Sharp, lancinating
- Reflex loss
- Sensory loss
- Smooth, fine skin
- Weakness

Diagnostic Tests
- EMG
- Somatosensory testing

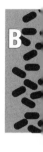

Pharmacologic Management
- Anticonvulsants (for stabbing, shocklike component)
  - Carbamazepine, 200–1600 mg/day PO
  - Phenytoin 300–500 mg/day PO
- Antidepressants
  - Amitriptyline, 25–150 mg/day PO
  - Doxepin 25–150 mg/day PO
  - Imipramine 20–100 mg/day PO
  - Trazodone 75–225 mg/day PO
- Local anesthesias
  - Lidocaine 5 mg/kg IV
  - Mexiletine 450–600 mg/day PO
  - Tocainide 20 mg/kg/day PO

Nonpharmacologic Management
- Acupuncture
- Distraction
- Hypnosis
- Relaxation and imagery
- TENS

Potential Problems
- Depression
- Fatigue
- Impaired mobility
- Impaired skin integrity
- Potential for injury

Pruritus

Definition
• An unpleasant sensation of the skin that initiates the desire to scratch

Etiology/Risk Factors
• Adenocarcinoma
• Advanced brain tumors
• Anemia
• Anxiety
• Carcinoid syndrome
• Dehydration
• Diabetes
• Hodgkin's disease
• Liver dysfunction
• Multiple myeloma
• Non-Hodgkin's lymphoma
• Opioids
• Polycythemia
• Renal dysfunction
• Stress
• Thyroid disease

Assessment
• Dryness of skin
• Erythema
• Excoriation
• Pustules
• Scab formation
• Scratch marks
• Skin condition
• Urticaria

Diagnostic Tests
• None

Pharmacologic Management

• Antihistamines (e.g., Periactin, Benadryl, Vistaril)
• Local, topical anesthetics

Nonpharmacologic Management

• Administer cool or tepid baths/showers
• Avoid alcohol
• Fluid intake of at least 3000 ml/day
• Keep humidity in room at 30–40%
• Keep room temperature cool
• Protect skin integrity (e.g., short nails, protective clothing)
• Use cutaneous stimulation
• Use relaxation techniques
• Use soothing substances in bath (e.g., starch, oatmeal)

Potential problems
• Anxiety
• Infection
• Insomnia
• Skin breakdown

Sedation

Definition
- The act of calming, usually by administration of a sedative

Etiology/Risk Factors
- Barbiturates
- Benzodiazepines
- Infectious processes
- Metabolic abnormalities
- Neurologic dysfunction (primary tumors, metastases)
- Opioids
- Phenothiazines
- Sleep deprivation

Assessment
- Decreased attention span
- Disorientation
- Drooping eyelids
- Sleepiness

Diagnostic Tests
- CT
- MRI

Pharmacologic Management
- Discontinue sedative drugs, if appropriate
- For opioid-induced sedation
  - Dextroamphetamine, 2.5–10 mg/day PO, in two doses at 8:00 A.M. and 12:00 noon
  - Methylphenidate, 5–10 mg/day, PO, in two doses at 8:00 A.M. and 12:00 noon
- Institute measures to reverse the metabolic causes of sedation

Nonpharmacologic Management
- Assistance with ADL
- Orientation activities (e.g., provision of calendar, clock)
- Safety precautions

Potential Problems
- Aspiration
- Fatigue
- Immobility
- Potential for injury
- Self-care deficit

Seizures

Definition
• A violent spasm or series of jerkings of the face, trunk, or extremities

Etiology/Risk Factors
• Infections
• Metabolic disorders (e.g., hypocalcemia, hypernatremia)
• Tumors (especially in frontal, parietal, and temporal lobes) and brain metastases

Assessment
• Headache
• Lethargy
• Mood alterations
• Myoclonic jerks

Diagnostic Tests
• CBC
• CT
• EEG
• MRI
• Serum electrolytes

Pharmacologic Management

• Carbamazepine, 600–1200 mg/day, PO, in two doses
• Filbamate, 1200–3600 mg/day, PO, in three doses
• Phenobarbital, 100–200 mg/day, PO, in one dose
• Phenytoin, 200–400 mg/day PO, in one dose
• Primidone, 750–1500 mg/day PO, in three doses
• Valproic acid, 1500–2000 mg/day PO, in three doses

Nonpharmacologic Management

• Avoid dangerous situations (e.g., driving a motor vehicle)
• Monitor plasma levels of antiseizure medications
• Radiation therapy (for tumors)
• Surgery (for tumors)

Potential Problems
• Depression
• Potential for injury
• Self-care deficit

Skin Desquamation: Dry

Definition
- The skin becomes dry and scaly owing to the destruction of the sebaceous glands in the radiation treatment field

Etiology/Risk Factors
- Radiation treatments to sensitive skin areas
  - Inflamed or infected skin
  - Skin with poor blood supply (backs of hands, tops and soles of feet, midline of back)
- Skin surfaces subject to friction and moisture (breasts, buttocks, axillae, groins, vulva)
- Skin traumatized by surgery or injury
- Smooth, thin skin (axillae, face, groins, perineum)

Assessment
- Pain
- Pruritis
- Skin assessment
  - Color
  - Moisture
  - Scaling
  - Temperature

Diagnostic Tests
- None

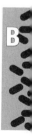

Pharmacologic Management
- Nonopioid analgesics

Nonpharmacologic Management
- Avoid applications of heat or cold
- Avoid oil-based creams, ointments, lotions
- Avoid shaving
- Avoid sun exposure
- Avoid tight clothing
- Keep skin dry (use a hair dryer if necessary)
- Meticulous skin care
- Optimal positioning
- Strict hand washing
- Use cornstarch to decrease friction

Potential Problems
- Infection
- Pain
- Pruritus

Skin Desquamation: Moist

Definition
- The skin develops blisters, and peeling of the epithelial layers of the skin is secondary to skin damage from radiation therapy

Etiology/Risk Factors
- Radiation treatments to sensitive skin areas
- Inflamed or infected skin
- Skin with poor blood supply (backs of hands, tops and soles of feet, midline of back)
- Skin surfaces subject to friction and moisture (breasts, buttocks, axillae, groins, vulva)
- Skin traumatized by surgery or injury
- Smooth, thin skin (axillae, face, groins, perineum)

Assessment
- Drainage: color, odor, amount, consistency
- Pain
- Pruritus
- Skin assessment
  - Color
  - Moisture
  - Scaling
  - Temperature

Diagnostic Test
- Culture

Pharmacologic Management
- Opioid analgesics
- Topical Aquaphor or aqueous lanolin

Nonpharmacologic Management
- Avoid shaving
- Avoid sun exposure
- Avoid tight clothing
- Keep skin dry (use a hair dryer if necessary)
- Meticulous skin care
- Optimal positioning
- Strict hand washing
- Use cornstarch to decrease friction
- Use wet dressings

Potential Problems
- Infection
- Pain
- Pruritus

Skin Lesions: Nonulcerating

Definition
• A pathologic change in tissue on the surface of the skin

Etiology/Risk Factors
• Breast
• Colon or rectum
• Kaposi's sarcoma
• Lung
• Lymphoma
• Malignant melanoma
• Ovary

Assessment
• Assessment of skin lesions
  • Configuration
  • Drainage
  • General characteristics
  • Location and distribution
  • Morphologic structure
  • Size
• Pruritus
• Skin assessment
  • Color
  • Edema
  • Lesions
  • Nodules
  • Scars
  • Vascularity

Diagnostic Tests
• Biopsy
• Culture

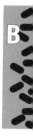

Pharmacologic Management

• Antihistamines
• Nonsteroidal antiinflammatory drugs

Nonpharmacologic Management

• Avoid pressure to the site
• Gentle skin care
• Protect skin from trauma
• Use dry dressings to protect the skin

Potential Problems
• Infection
• Pain

Skin Lesions: Ulcerating

Definition
- A lesion on the surface of the skin caused by superficial loss of tissue, usually with inflammation

Etiology/Risk Factors
- Breast
- Colon or rectum
- Kaposi's sarcoma
- Lung
- Lymphoma
- Malignant melanoma
- Ovary

Assessment
- Assessment of skin lesions
  - Configuration
  - Drainage
  - General characteristics
  - Location and distribution
  - Morphologic structure
  - Size
- Pruritus
- Skin assessment
  - Color
  - Edema
  - Lesions
  - Nodules
  - Scars
  - Vascularity

Diagnostic Tests
- Biopsy
- Culture

Pharmacologic Management
- Antihistamines
- Nonopioid analgesics
- Opioid analgesics

Nonpharmacologic Management
- Avoid cross-contamination
- Débride wound as necessary
- Gentle skin care
- High-protein, high-calorie diet
- Irrigate wound
- Sterile, nonadherent dressings
- Absorbent pads to control drainage
- Agents to achieve hemostasis
- Agents to control odor (balsam of Peru)

Potential Problems
- Infection
- Pain

Thrombocytopenia

Definition

- An abnormal decrease in the number of circulating platelets that may result in bleeding or hemorrhage

Etiology/Risk Factors

- Allergic reactions
- Chemotherapy
- CLL
- Hypersplenism
- Lymphoma
- Tumor invasion of bone marrow

Assessment

- Change in mental status
- Dizziness
- Ecchymosis
- Epistaxis
- Hematemesis
- Hematomas
- Hematuria
- Petechiae
- Prolonged bleeding
- Vital sign changes

Diagnostic Tests

- Testing for occult blood (urine, stool, emesis)
- Platelet count

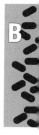

Pharmacologic Management

- Platelet transfusions

Nonpharmacologic Management

- Avoid injections
- Avoid invasive procedures
- Avoid sharp objects
- Bowel regimen to prevent constipation
- Prevent trauma to rectal mucosa (e.g., avoid enemas, rectal temperatures)
- Promote rest and comfort
- Soft, bland diet
- Soft toothbrush

Potential Problems

- Anxiety
- Fatigue
- Hemorrhage
- Potential for injury
- Self-care deficit

Urinary Retention

Definition
- Abrupt cessation of urine output through the urethra

Etiology/Risk Factors
- Infection
- Opioids
- Tumor obstruction

Assessment
- Fever (sometimes)
- Insidious onset
- Oliguria
- Pain
- Sensation of bladder fullness

Diagnostic Tests
- Abdominal CT
- Abdominal radiography
- Bladder palpation
- Serum BUN and creatinine
- Urinalysis

Pharmacologic Management
- None

Nonpharmacologic Management
- Indwelling Foley catheter
- Intermittent bladder catheterization
- Urinary diversion

Potential Problems
- Alteration in sexual functioning
- Altered body image
- Infection
- Pain

Vaginal Dryness

Definition
• Decreased lubrication of the female genital canal extending from the uterus to the vulva

Etiology/Risk Factors
• Chemotherapy
• Gynecologic malignancies
• Gynecologic surgery
• Pelvic radiation

Assessment
• History
  • Bleeding
  • Discharge
  • Dyspareunia
  • Odor
  • Pain
  • Pruritus
  • Soreness
• Vaginal examination
  • Decrease in vaginal size
  • Erythema
  • Fibrosis/stenosis
  • Swelling
  • Tone/lubrication

Diagnostic Tests
• None

Pharmacologic Management

• Estrogen creams and suppositories

Nonpharmacologic Management

• Cool compresses to perineal area
• Female-on-top position for intercourse
• Psychological counseling
• Systematic desensitization
• Use of water-soluble lubricant

Potential Problems
• Altered body image
• Anxiety
• Depression
• Pain
• Pruritus

Weight Gain

Definition
- Increase in body weight above ideal body weight

Etiology/Risk Factors
- Androgens
- Anxiety
- Decreased mobility
- Depression
- Steroids
- Tamoxifen

Assessment
- Activity pattern
- Current weight
- Depression
- Dietary history
- Family history of obesity

Diagnostic Tests
- CBC
- Serum albumin
- Serum cholesterol
- Serum estradiol
- Serum triglycerides
- Total protein

Pharmacologic Management
- None

Nonpharmacologic Management
- Consult with a dietician
- Diet plan
- Exercise program
- Referral to appropriate support groups (e.g., Weight Watchers, Overeaters Anonymous)

Potential Problems
- Decreased mobility
- Decreased social interaction
- Depression
- Fatigue

Weight Loss

Definition
· Decrease in body weight below ideal weight

Etiology/Risk Factors
· Anxiety
· Biologic therapy
· Cancer diagnosis
· Chemotherapy
· Depression
· Metastatic disease
· Pain
· Radiation therapy
· Surgery

Assessment
· Alterations in bowel elimination (e.g., constipation, diarrhea)
· Condition of oral cavity
· Current weight
· Mood disturbance

Diagnostic Tests
· Anthropometry
· CBC
· Iron-binding capacity
· Serum albumin
· Serum cholesterol
· Serum triglycerides
· Total protein

Pharmacologic Management

•   Enteral nutritional supplements
•   High-protein, high-calorie diet
•   Nutritional supplements (e.g., Isocal, Ensure, Ensure Plus, Carnation Instant Breakfast)
•   Total parenteral nutrition

Nonpharmacologic Management

•   Appropriate referrals (e.g., Meals on Wheels)
•   Consult with dietician
•   Dental consult
•   Eliminate nonnutritious foods
•   Exercise program
•   Oral care regimen
•   Small, frequent meals

Potential Problems
· Decreased mobility
· Depression
· Fatigue
· Infection
· Self-care deficit

Xerostomia

Definition
- Dryness of the mucous membranes of the oral cavity secondary to inadequate or absent saliva production

Etiology/Risk Factors
- Antihistamines
- Dehydration
- Infection
- Radiation therapy

Assessment
- Duration of xerostomia
- Oral assessment
- Status of teeth and gums

Diagnostic Tests
- None

Pharmacologic Management
- Fluoride gel on a carrier molded to fit the contour of the mouth

Nonpharmacologic Management
- Artificial saliva
- Avoid alcohol and tobacco
- Avoid chemical and thermal irritants
- Dental consult
- Lubricate lips
- Maintain fluid intake throughout the day
- Routine oral care
- Have patient suck on substances that stimulate saliva production

Potential Problems
- Dental caries
- Infection
- Nutritional deficit
- Pain

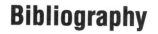

Bibliography

Alopecia

Tollenaar, R. A., Liefers, G. J., Repelaer van Driel, O. J., & van de Velde, C. J. (1994). Scalp cooling has no place in the prevention of alopecia in adjuvant chemotherapy for breast cancer. *European Journal of Cancer, 1994, 30A*(10), 1448–1453.

Anemia

Mohandas, K., & Aledort, L. (1995). Transfusion requirements, risks, and costs for patients with malignancy. *Transfusion, 35*(5), 427–430.

Rieger, P. T., & Haeuber, D. (1995). A new approach to managing chemotherapy-related anemia: Nursing implications of epoetin alfa. *Oncology Nursing Forum, 22*(1), 71–81.

Anorexia

Nelson, K. A., Walsh, D., & Sheehan, F. A. (1994). The cancer anorexia-cachexia syndrome. *Journal of Clinical Oncology, 12*(1), 213–225.

Parnes, H. L., & Aisner, J. (1992). Protein calorie malnutrition and cancer therapy. *Drug Safety, 7*(6), 404–416.

Pisters, P. W., & Pearlstone, D. B. (1993). Protein and amino acid metabolism in cancer cachexia: Investigative techniques and therapeutic interventions. *Critical Reviews in Clinical Laboratory Sciences, 30*(3), 223–272.

Anxiety

Genuis, M. L. (1995). The use of hypnosis in helping cancer patients control anxiety, pain, and emesis: A review of recent empirical studies. *American Journal of Clinical Hypnosis, 37*(4), 316–325.

Harrison, J., & Maguire, P. (1994). Predictors of psychiatric morbidity in cancer patients. *British Journal of Psychiatry, 165*(5), 593–598.

Trijsburg, R. W., van Knippenberg, F. C., & Rijpma, S. E. (1992). Effects of psychological treatment on cancer patients. A critical review. *Psychosomatic Medicine, 4*(4), 489–517.

Constipation

Bruera, E., Suarez-Almazor, M., Velasco, A., Bertolino, M., MacDonald, S. M., & Hanson, J. (1994). The assessment of constipation in terminal cancer patients admitted to a palliative care unit: A retrospective review. *Journal of Pain and Symptom Management, 9*(8), 515–519.

Gattuso, J. M., & Kamm, M. A. (1993). Review article: The management of constipation in adults. *Alimentary Pharmacology and Therapeutics, 7*(5), 487–500.

Wiseman, L. R., & Faulds, D. (1994). Cisapride. An updated review of its pharmacology and therapeutic efficacy as a prokinetic agent in gastrointestinal motility disorders. *Drugs, 47*(1), 116–152.

Cystitis

Levenback, C., Eifel, P. J., Burke, T. W., Morris, M., & Gershenson, D. M. (1994). Hemorrhagic cystitis following radiotherapy for stage Ib cancer of the cervix. *Gynecologic Oncology, 55*(2), 206–210.

deVries, C. R., & Freiha, F. S. (1990). Hemorrhagic cystitis: A review. *Journal of Urology, 143*(1), 1–9.

Depression

Fincannon, J. L. (1995). Analysis of psychiatric referrals and interventions in an oncology population. *Oncology Nursing Forum, 22*(1), 87–92.

Haig, R. A. (1992). Management of depression in patients with advanced cancer. *Medical Journal of Australia, 156*(7), 499–503.

Massie, M. J., Gagnon, P., & Holland, J. C. (1994). Depression and suicide in patients with cancer. *Journal of Pain and Symptom Management, 9*(5), 325–340.

Massie, M. J., & Holland, J. C. (1990). Depression and the cancer patient. *Journal of Clinical Psychiatry, 51*(Suppl.), 12–17.

McGee, R., Williams, S., & Elwood, M. (1994). Depression and the development of cancer: A meta-analysis. *Social Science and Medicine, 38*(1), 187–192.

Diarrhea

Mercadante, S. (1995). Diarrhea in terminally ill patients: Pathophysiology and treatment. *Journal of Pain and Symptom Management, 10*(4), 298–309.

Dysphagia

Boyce, G. A. (1990). Palliation of malignant esophageal obstruction. *Dysphagia, 5*(4), 220–226.

Dyspnea

Farncombe, M., Chater, S., & Gillin, A. (1994). The use of nebulized opioids for breathlessness: A chart review. *Palliative Medicine, 8*(4), 306–312.

Extravasation

Boyle, D. M., & Engelking, C. (1995). Vesicant extravasation: Myths and realities. *Oncology Nursing Forum, 22*(1), 57–67.

Gault, D. T. (1993). Extravasation injuries. *British Journal of Plastic Surgery, 46*(2), 91–96.

Fatigue

Blondel-Hill, E., & Shafran, S. D. (1993). Treatment of the chronic fatigue syndrome. A review and practical guide. *Drugs, 46*(4), 639–651.

Downey, D. C. (1992). Fatigue syndromes: New thoughts and reinterpretation of previous data. *Medical Hypotheses, 39*(2), 185–190.

Fox, D. S. (1994). Chronic fatigue syndrome: A review and practical guide. *Journal of the American Academy of Nurse Practitioners, 6*(12), 565–570.

Hypoxemia

Shigeoka, J. W., & Stults, B. M. (1992). Home oxygen therapy under Medicare. A primer. *Western Journal of Medicine, 156*(1), 39–44.

Impotence

Crasilneck, H. B. (1992). The use of hypnosis in the treatment of impotence. *Psychiatric Medicine, 10*(1), 67–75.

Dow, J. A., Gluck, R. W., Golimbu, M., Weinberg, G. I., & Morales, P. (1991). Multiphasic diagnostic evaluation of arteriogenic, venogenic, and sinusoidogenic impotency. Value of noninvasive tests compared with penile duplex ultrasonography. *Urology, 38*(5), 402–407.

Filiberti, A., Audisio, R. A., Gangeri, L., Baldini, M. T., Tamburini, M., Belli, F., Parc, R., & Leo, E. (1994). Prevalence of sexual dysfunction in male cancer patients treated with rectal excision and coloanal anastomosis. *European Journal of Surgical Oncology, 20*(1), 43–46.

Singer, P. A., Tasch, E. S., Stocking, C., Rubin, S., Siegler, M., & Weichselbaum, R. (1991). Sex or survival: Trade-offs between quality and quantity of life. *Journal of Clinical Oncology, 9*(2), 328–334.

Infection: Eyes

Snyder, R. W., & Glasser, D. B. (1994). Antibiotic therapy for ocular infection. *Western Journal of Medicine, 161*(6), 579–584.

Thomas, R. K., & Melton, N. R. (1992). A review of common ophthalmic antibacterial and corticosteroid-antibacterial combination drugs. *Optometry Clinics, 2*(4), 45–57.

Infection: Genitourinary Tract

Bartlett, R. C., Zern, D. A., Ratkiewicz, I., & Tetreault, J. Z. (1994). Reagent strip screening for sediment abnormalities identified by automated microscopy in urine from patients suspected to have urinary tract disease. *Archives of Pathology and Laboratory Medicine, 118*(11), 1096–1101.

Bishop, M. C. (1994). Urosurgical management of urinary tract infection. *Journal of Antimicrobial Chemotherapy, 33*(Suppl. A), 75–91.

Hooton, T. M., & Stam, W. E. (1991). Management of acute uncomplicated urinary tract infection in adults. *Medical Clinics of North America, 75*(2), 339–357.

Infection: Mucous Membranes

Scully, C., el-Kabir, M., & Samaranayake, L. P. (1994). *Candida* and oral candidosis: A review. *Critical Reviews in Oral Biology and Medicine, 5*(2), 125–157.

Shillitoe, E. J. (1991). Relationship of viral infection to malignancies. *Current Opinion in Dentistry, 1*(4), 398–403.

Infection: Respiratory Tract

Hanna, J. W., Reed, J. C., & Choplin, R. H. (1991). Pleural infections: A clinical-radiologic review. *Journal of Thoracic Imaging, 6*(3), 68–79.

Levine, S. J. (1992). An approach to the diagnosis of pulmonary infections in immunosuppressed patients. *Seminars in Respiratory Infections, 7*(2), 81–95.

Infection: Skin

Chren, M. M., Lazarus, H. M., Bickers, D. R., & Landefeld, C. S. (1993). Rashes in immunocompromised cancer patients. The diagnostic yield of skin biopsy and its effects on therapy. *Archives of Dermatology, 129*(2), 175–181.

Goldenheim, P. D. (1993). An appraisal of povidone-iodine and wound healing. *Postgraduate Medical Journal, 69*(Suppl. 3), S97–S105.

Jewell, M. E., & Sweet, D. E. (1994). Oral and dermatologic manifestations of HIV infection. *Postgraduate Medicine, 96*(5), 105–108, 111, 114–116.

Novakova, I. R., Donnelly, J. P., & De Pauw, B. (1993). Potential sites of infection that develop in febrile neutropenic patients. *Leukemia and Lymphoma, 10*(6), 461–467.

Strauss, F. G., Holmes, D. L., Nortman, D. F., & Friedman, S. (1993). Hypertonic saline compresses: Therapy for complicated exit-site infections. *Advances in Peritoneal Dialysis, 9,* 248–250.

Valainis, G. T. (1994). Dermatologic manifestations of nosocomial infections. *Infectious Disease Clinics of North America, 8*(3), 617–635.

Zalla, M. J., Su, W. P., & Fransway, A. F. (1992). Dermatologic manifestations of human immunodeficiency virus infection. *Mayo Clinic Proceedings, 67*(11), 1089–1108.

Infection: Systemic

Au, E., & Ang, P. T. (1993). Management of chemotherapy-induced neutropenic sepsis—combination of cephalosporin and aminoglycoside. *Annals of the Academy of Medicine, Singapore, 22*(3), 319–322.

Barriere, S. L., & Lowry, S. F. (1995). An overview of mortality risk prediction in sepsis. *Critical Care Medicine, 23*(2), 376–393.

Curtin, J. P., Hoskins, W. J., Rubin, S. C., Jones, W. B., Hakes, T. B., Markman, M. M., Reichman, B., Almadrones, L., & Lewis, J. L., Jr. (1991). Chemotherapy-induced neutropenia and fever in patients receiving cisplatin-based chemotherapy for ovarian malignancy. *Gynecologic Oncology, 40*(1), 17–20.

Eastridge, B. J., & Lefor, A. T. (1995). Complications of indwelling venous access devices in cancer patients. *Journal of Clinical Oncology, 13*(1), 233–238.

Raad, I., Davis, S., Khan, A., Tarrand, J., Elting, L., & Bodey, G. P. (1992). Impact of central venous catheter removal on the recurrence of catheter-related coagulase-negative staphylococcal bacteremia. *Infection Control and Hospital Epidemiology, 13*(4), 215–221.

Infertility

Dow, K. H. (1995). A review of late effects of cancer in women. *Seminars in Oncology Nursing, 11*(2), 128–136.

Reichman, B. S., & Green, K. B. (1994). Breast cancer in young women: Effect of chemotherapy on ovarian function, fertility, and birth defects. *Monographs/National Cancer Institute,* (16), 125–129.

Insomnia

Ancoli-Israel, S., & Kripke, D. F. (1991). Prevalent sleep problems in the aged. *Biofeedback and Self Regulation, 16*(4), 349–359.

Becker, P. M., & Jamieson, A. O. (1992). Common sleep disorders in the elderly: Diagnosis and treatment. *Geriatrics, 47*(3), 41–42, 45–48, 51–52.

Morin, C. M., Culbert, J. P., & Schwartz, S. M. (1994). Nonpharmacological interventions for insomnia: A meta-analysis of treatment efficacy. *American Journal of Psychiatry, 151*(8), 1172–1180.

Thorpy, M. J. (1990). Classification of sleep disorders. *Journal of Clinical Neurophysiology, 7*(1), 67–81.

Lymphedema

Brennan, M. J. (1992). Lymphedema following the surgical treatment of breast cancer: A review of pathophysiology and treatment. *Journal of Pain and Symptom Management, 7*(2), 110–116.

Bunce, I. H., Mirolo, B. R., Hennessy, J. M., Ward, L. C., & Jones, L. C. (1994). Post-mastectomy lymphoedema treatment and measurement. *Medical Journal of Australia, 161*(2), 125–128.

Granda, C. (1994). Nursing management of patients with lymphedema associated with breast cancer therapy. *Cancer Nursing, 17*(3), 229–235.

Williams, A. E. (1992). Management of lymphoedema: A community-based approach. *British Journal of Nursing, 1*(8), 383, 385–387.

Mucositis

Barker, G., Loftus, L., Cuddy, P., & Barker, B. (1991). The effects of sucralfate suspension and diphenhydramine syrup plus kaolin-pectin on radiotherapy-induced mucositis. *Oral Surgery, Oral Medicine, Oral Pathology, 71*(3), 288–293.

Nausea and Vomiting: Acute

Genuis, M. L. (1995). The use of hypnosis in helping cancer patients control anxiety, pain, and emesis: A review of recent empirical studies. *American Journal of Clinical Hypnosis, 37*(4), 316–325.

Gin, T. (1994). Recent advances in the understanding and management of postoperative nausea and vomiting. *Annals of the Academy of Medicine, Singapore, 23*(6, Suppl.), 114–119.

Gralla, R. J. (1993). Current issues in the management of nausea and vomiting. *Annals of Oncology, 4*(Suppl. 3), S3–S7.

Perez, A. (1995). Review of the preclinical pharmacology and comparative efficacy of 5-hydroxytryptamine-3 receptor antagonists for chemotherapy-induced emesis. *Journal of Clinical Oncology, 13*(4), 1036–1043.

Perez, E. A., & Gandara, D. R. (1992). Advances in the control of chemotherapy-induced emesis. *Annals of Oncology, 3*(Suppl. 3), 47–50.

Roberts, J. T., & Priestman, T. J. (1993). A review of ondansetron in the management of radiotherapy-induced emesis. *Oncology, 50*(3), 173–179.

Rousseau, P. (1995). Antiemetic therapy in adults with terminal disease: A brief review. *American Journal of Hospice and Palliative Care, 12*(1), 13–18.

Soukop, M. (1994). Clinical experience with intravenous granisetron. *Anti-Cancer Drugs, 5*(3), 281–286.

Nausea and Vomiting: Anticipatory

Andrykowski, M. A. (1990). The role of anxiety in the development of anticipatory nausea in cancer chemotherapy: A review and synthesis. *Psychosomatic Medicine, 52*(4), 458–475.

Oral Candidiasis

van der Bijl, P., & Arendorf, T. M. (1993). Itraconazole and fluconazole in oropharyngeal candidiasis. *Annals of Dentistry, 52*(2), 12–16.

Fotos, P. G., & Ray, T. L. (1994). Oral and perioral candidosis. *Seminars in Dermatology, 13*(2), 118–124.

Jeganathan, S., & Chan, Y. C. (1992). Immunodiagnosis in oral candidiasis. A review. *Oral Surgery, Oral Medicine, Oral Pathology, 74*(4), 451–454.

Scully, C., el-Kabir, M., & Samaranayake, L. P. (1994). Candida and oral candidosis: A review. *Critical Reviews in Oral Biology and Medicine, 5*(2), 125–157.

Oral Herpes Infection

Blondeau, J. M., & Embil, J. A. (1990). Herpes simplex virus infection: What to look for. What to do! *Journal/Canadian Dental Association. Journal de l'Association Dentaire Canadienne* (Ottawa), *56*(8), 785–787.

Elliott, S. Y., Kerns, F. T., & Kitchen, L. W. (1993). Herpes esophagitis in immunocompetent adults: Report of two cases and review of the literature. *West Virginia Medical Journal, 89*(5), 188–190.

Rayani, S. A., Nimmo, C. J., Frighetto, L., Martinusen, S. M., Nickoloff, D. M., Reece, D. E., & Jewesson, P. J. (1994). Implementation and evaluation of a standardized herpes simplex virus prophylaxis protocol on a leukemia/bone marrow transplant unit. *Annals of Pharmacotherapy, 28*(7–8), 852–856.

Reichart, P. A. (1991). Oral manifestations of

recently described viral infections, including AIDS. *Current Opinion in Dentistry, 1*(4), 377–383.

Pain: Acute Postoperative

Goodchild, C. S. (1993). Acute postoperative pain: Logical treatment by drug combinations. *British Journal of Theatre Nursing, 2*(12), 15–19.

Jurf, J. B., & Nirschl, A. L. (1993). Acute postoperative pain management: A comprehensive review and update. *Critical Care Nursing Quarterly, 16*(1), 8–25.

Mather, C. M., & Ready, L. B. (1994). Management of acute pain. *British Journal of Hospital Medicine, 51*(3), 85–88.

Musgrave, C. F. (1990). Acute postoperative pain: The cause and the care. *Journal of Post Anesthesia Nursing, 5*(5), 329–337.

Pain: Bone Metastasis

Lewington, V. J. (1993). Targeted radionuclide therapy for bone metastases. *European Journal of Nuclear Medicine, 20*(1), 66–74.

Pain: Neuropathic

Ochoa, J. L. (1994). Pain mechanisms in neuropathy. *Current Opinion in Neurology, 7*(5), 407–414.

Woolf, C. J. (1993). The pathophysiology of peripheral neuropathic pain—abnormal peripheral input and abnormal central processing. *Acta Neurochirurgica, Supplementum.* (Wien), *58,* 125–130.

Pain: Visceral

Ness, T. J., & Gebhart, G. F. (1990). Visceral pain: A review of experimental studies. *Pain, 41*(2), 167–234.

Talley, N. J. (1992). Review article: 5-Hydroxytryptamine agonists and antagonists in the modulation of gastrointestinal motility and sensation: Clinical implications. *Alimentary Pharmacology and Therapeutics, 6*(3), 273–289.

Peripheral Neuropathy

Cohen, J. A., & Gross, K. F. (1990). Peripheral neuropathy: Causes and management in the elderly. *Geriatrics, 45*(2), 21–26, 31–34.

Ochoa, J. L. (1994). Pain mechanisms in neuropathy. *Current Opinion in Neurology, 7*(5), 407–414.

Sedation

Macnab, A. J., Levine, M., Glick, N., Susak, L., & Baker-Brown, G. (1991). A research tool for measurement of recovery from sedation: The Vancouver Sedative Recovery Scale. *Journal of Pediatric Surgery, 26*(11), 1263–1267.

Waldman, H. J. (1994). Centrally acting skeletal muscle relaxants and associated drugs. *Journal of Pain and Symptom Management, 9*(7), 434–441.

Westcott, C. (1995). The sedation of patients in intensive care units: A nursing review. *Intensive and Critical Care Nursing, 11*(1), 26–31.

Seizures

Agbi, C. B., & Bernstein, M. (1993). Seizure prophylaxis for brain tumour patients. Brief

review and guide for family physicians. *Canadian Family Physician, 39,* 1153–1156, 1159–1160, 1163–1164.

Hagmeyer, K. O., Mauro, L. S., & Mauro, V. F. (1993). Meperidine-related seizures associated with patient-controlled analgesia pumps. *Annals of Pharmacotherapy, 27*(1), 29–32.

Henneman, P. L., DeRoos, F., & Lewis, R. J. (1994). Determining the need for admission in patients with new-onset seizures. *Annals of Emergency Medicine, 24*(6), 1108–1114.

Patsalos, P. N., & Sander, J. W. (1994). Newer antiepileptic drugs. Towards an improved risk-benefit ratio. *Drug Safety, 11*(1), 37–67.

Shin, C., & McNamara, J. O. (1994). Mechanism of epilepsy. *Annual Review of Medicine, 45* 379–389.

So, N. K. (1993). Recurrence, remission, and relapse of seizures. *Cleveland Clinic Journal of Medicine, 60*(6), 439–444.

Skin Desquamation: Dry

Ross, E. V. (1991). Ichthyosiform scaling secondary to megavoltage radiotherapy. *Cutis, 48*(1), 59–60.

Skin Lesions

Kerdel, F. A. (1993). Inflammatory ulcers. *Journal of Dermatologic Surgery and Oncology, 19*(8), 772–778.

Kiritsy, C. P., Lynch, A. B., & Lynch, S. E. (1993). Role of growth factors in cutaneous wound healing: A review. *Critical Reviews in Oral Biology and Medicine, 1993, 4*(5), 729–760.

Margolis, D. J., & Lewis, V. L. (1995). A literature assessment of the use of miscellaneous topical agents, growth factors, and skin equivalents for the treatment of pressure ulcers. *Dermatologic Surgery, 21*(2), 145–148.

Phillips, T. J. (1994). Chronic cutaneous ulcers: Etiology and epidemiology. *Journal of Investigative Dermatology, 102*(6), 38S–41S.

Yarkony, G. M. (1994). Pressure ulcers: A review. *Archives of Physical Medicine and Rehabilitation, 75*(8), 908–917.

Thrombocytopenia

Baughman, R. P., Lower, E. E., Flessa, H. C., & Tollerud, D. J. (1993). Thrombocytopenia in the intensive care unit. *Chest, 104*(4), 1243–1247.

Bick, R. L. (1992). Coagulation abnormalities in malignancy: A review. *Seminars in Thrombosis and Hemostasis, 18*(4), 353–372.

Kelsey, H. C. (1992). An audit of the use of platelet concentrates in the prophylaxis of thrombocytopenic haemorrhage in a large haematology unit. *Blood Coagulation and Fibrinolysis, 3*(5), 647–649.

Metz, J., McGrath, K. M., Copperchini, M. L., Haeusler, M., Haysom, H. E., Gibson, P. R., Millar, R. J., Babarczy, A., Ferris, L., & Grigg, A. P. (1995). Appropriateness of transfusions of red cells, platelets and fresh frozen plasma. An audit in a tertiary care teaching hospital. *Medical Journal of Australia, 162*(11), 572–573, 576–577.

Mueller-Eckhardt, C., Kiefel, V., & Santoso, S. (1990). Review and update of platelet alloantigen systems. *Transfusion Medicine Reviews, 4*(2), 98–109.

Shulkin, D. J., Fox, K. R., & Stadtmauer, E. A. (1992). Guidelines for prophylactic platelet transfusions: Need for a concurrent outcomes management system. *Quality Review Bulletin, 18*(12), 477–479.

Simsek, S., & von dem Borne, A. E. (1994). Molecular genetics of human platelet antigens. *Infusionstherapie und Transfusionsmedizin, 21*(Suppl. 3), 29–33.

Urinary Retention

Feinberg, M. (1993). The problems of anticholinergic adverse effects in older patients. *Drugs and Aging, 3*(4), 335–348.

Freeman, R., & Miyawaki, E. (1993). The treatment of autonomic dysfunction. *Journal of Clinical Neurophysiology, 10*(1), 61–82.

Hastie, K. J., Dickinson, A. J., Ahmad, R., & Moisey, C. U. (1990). Acute retention of urine: Is trial without catheter justified? *Journal of the Royal College of Surgeons of Edinburgh, 35*(4), 225–227.

Taub, H. C., & Stein, M. (1994). Bladder distention therapy for symptomatic relief of frequency and urgency: A ten-year review. *Urology, 43*(1), 36–39.

Vaginal Dryness

Sarrel, P. M. (1990). Ovarian hormones and the circulation. *Maturitas, 12*(3), 287–298.

Weight Gain

Demark-Wahnefried, W., Winer, E. P., & Rimer, B. K. (1993). Why women gain weight with adjuvant chemotherapy for breast cancer. *Journal of Clinical Oncology, 11*(7), 1418–1429.

Weight Loss

Heys, S. D., Park, K. G., Garlick, P. J., & Eremin, O. (1992). Nutrition and malignant disease: Implications for surgical practice. *British Journal of Surgery, 79*(7), 614–623.

Morley, J. E., & Kraenzle, D. (1994). Causes of weight loss in a community nursing home. *Journal of the American Geriatrics Society, 42*(6), 583–585.

Parnes, H. L., & Aisner, J. (1992). Protein calorie malnutrition and cancer therapy. *Drug Safety, 7*(6), 404–416.

Pisters, P. W., & Pearlstone, D. B. (1993). Protein and amino acid metabolism in cancer cachexia: Investigative techniques and therapeutic interventions. *Critical Reviews in Clinical Laboratory Sciences, 30*(3), 223–272.

Xerostomia

Epstein, J. B., Stevenson-Moore, P., & Scully, C. (1992). Management of xerostomia. *Journal/Canadian Dental Association. Journal de L'Association Dentaire Canadienne* (Ottawa), *58*(2), 140–143.

Semba, S. E., Mealey, B. L., & Hallmon, W. W. (1994). The head and neck radiotherapy patient: Part 1—Oral manifestations of radiation therapy. *Compendium, 15*(2), 250, 252–260.

Wiseman, L. R., & Faulds, D. (1995). Oral pilocarpine: A review of its pharmacological properties and clinical potential in xerostomia. *Drugs, 49*(1), 143–155.

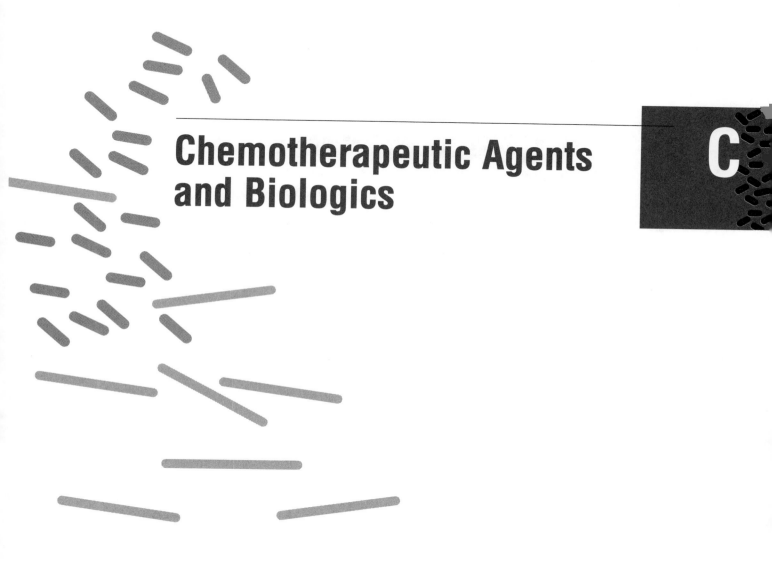

Chemotherapeutic Agents and Biologics

C

Aldesleukin · Interleukin-2, Proleukin, T-cell growth factor, Teceleukin

Drug Classification
Immunoregulating agent

Mechanism
- Stimulates activated T-cell growth and differentiation
- Proliferation and immunoglobulin production in B cells
- Macrophage cytotoxic activity
- Generation of LAK activity

Administration
- SC, IM, IV push, IV infusion, intraperitoneal, intrahepatic, intrapleural, intraventricular

Therapeutic Use
- Bladder
- Colorectal
- Head and neck
- Hodgkin's disease
- Leptomeningeal
- Lung
- Malignant melanoma
- NHL
- Ovarian
- Renal cell
- Stomach

Usual Dose and Schedule
- Renal cell: 600,000 IU/kg per dose as a 15-minute IV infusion q8h for 14 doses

Side Effects/Toxicities
- Anemia
- Atrial arrhythmias
- Capillary leak syndrome
- Confusion
- Delirium
- Diarrhea
- Flulike syndrome
- Local skin inflammation
- MI
- Nausea and vomiting
- Neutropenia
- Nephrotoxicity
- Thrombocytopenia
- Transient somnolence

Special Considerations
- Severe hypotension can occur with higher doses

Altretamine · Hexalen, Hexamethylmelamine

Drug classification
Alkylating agent

Mechanism
- Exact cytotoxic mechanism of action unknown
- Breakdown of metabolic by-product to formaldehyde may mediate cytotoxicity
- Inhibits incorporation of nucleotides into DNA and RNA

Administration
- PO, IV (investigational formulation)

Therapeutic Use
- Breast
- Bronchogenic carcinoma
- Cervical
- Childhood leukemias
- Lymphomas
- NHL
- Ovarian

Usual Dose and Schedule
- Single agent: 4–12 mg/kg/day
- Advanced ovarian cancer: 260 mg/m^2/day administered in 4 doses for 14–21 days of a 28-day treatment cycle
- Combination regimen: 150 mg/m^2 for 14 days of a 28-day cycle

Side Effects/Toxicities
- Agitation
- Abdominal cramps
- Anorexia
- Ataxia
- Confusion
- Depression
- Diarrhea
- Hallucinations
- Leukopenia
- Loss of deep tendon reflexes
- Nausea
- Paresthesias
- Parkinson-like symptoms
- Peripheral neuropathy
- Petit mal–type seizures
- Skin rash
- Thrombocytopenia
- Vomiting

Special Considerations
- May cause severe orthostatic hypotension when administered with MAO inhibitors

Aminoglutethimide · Cytadren, Elipten, Orimeten

Drug Classification
Nonsteroidal inhibitor of corticosteroid biosynthesis

Mechanism
- Binds to cytochrome P_{450} enzymes, blocking biosynthesis of corticosteroids
- Blocks conversion of androgens to estrogens
- Causes a chemical adrenalectomy

Administration
- Oral

Therapeutic Use
- Adrenocortical carcinoma
- Hormonally responsive breast cancer
- Prostate
- Symptomatic palliation in Cushing's disease

Usual Dose and Schedule

- For adrenal suppression: 750–1500 mg/day

Side Effects/Toxicities
- Ataxia
- Blurred vision
- Dizziness
- Elevated LFTs
- Facial flushing
- Hyponatremia
- Lethargy
- Maculopapular rash
- Mild vertigo
- Nausea and vomiting
- Postural hypotension
- Periorbital edema
- Somnolence

Special Considerations
- Avoid taking antacid tablets within 2 hours of taking enteric coated tablet
- 20–50% of patients require mineralocorticoid replacement (fludrocortisone, 0.1 mg/day or 3 times a week)

Amsacrine · Acridinyl anisidide, AMSA, Amsidine, *m*-AMSA

Drug Classification
Acridine derivative

Mechanism
- Intercalates between DNA base pairs
- Inhibits DNA synthesis
- Induces protein-linked DNA strand breaks

Administration
- Slow IV infusion, PO (investigational)

Therapeutic Use
- ALL (pediatric)
- ANLL (adult and pediatric)
- Advanced ovarian cancer
- Lymphoma
- Neuroblastoma

Usual Dose and Schedule
- Single agent: 120 mg/m^2 IV over 1–2 hours in 500 ml 5% dextrose and water for 5 days
- Combination regimen: 100 mg/m^2 IV over 1–2 hours in 500 ml 5% dextrose and water on days 7, 8, and 9

Side Effects/Toxicities
- Alopecia
- Anorexia
- Cardiac arrest
- Cholestasis
- Diarrhea
- Dizziness
- Congestive heart failure
- Elevation in serum alkaline phosphatase
- Extravasation
- Headache
- Leukopenia
- Malaise
- Mucositis
- Nausea and vomiting
- Peripheral neuropathy
- Phlebitis
- Seizures
- Skin rash

Special Considerations
- Acute ventricular arrhythmias are associated with rapid, highly concentrated infusions and/or hypokalemia
- Use a minimal infusion volume of 500 ml to reduce phlebitis
- May produce additive cardiotoxicity in patients who have received an anthracycline
- Solution physically incompatible with sodium chloride

L-Asparaginase · Crasnitin, Elspar

Drug Classification
Antitumor enzyme

Mechanism
- Acts indirectly to inhibit protein synthesis in tumor cells that are dependent on exogenous asparaginase
- Inhibition of DNA and RNA synthesis

Administration
- IM, slow IV push (over 30 minutes)

Therapeutic Use
- ALL

Usual Dose and Schedule

- Combination regimen: 1000 IU/kg/day IV × 10 days or 6000 IU/m^2/day IM for 9 injections every third day, starting the fourth day after cytotoxic therapy

Side Effects/Toxicities
- Acute pancreatitis
- Anaphylaxis
- Anemia
- Anorexia
- Depression
- Disorientation
- Hallucinations
- Hepatotoxicity
- Hypersensitivity reactions
- Lethargy
- Malaise
- Nausea and vomiting
- Somnolence
- Recent memory loss

Special Considerations
- Skin testing is recommended before L-asparaginase administration
- Be prepared to treat anaphylaxis
- May increase vincristine toxicity if given concurrently with or immediately before

Bacillus Calmette-Guérin · BCG, TheraCys, Tice

Drug Classification
Immunoaugmenting agent

Mechanism
· Exact mechanism unknown

Administration
· Intravesicular

Therapeutic Use
· Urinary bladder

Usual Dose and Schedule

· Three vials of TheraCys (27 mg BCG/vial) intravesically once a week for 6 weeks

Side Effects/Toxicities
· Dysuria
· Hematuria
· Urinary frequency
· Urinary tract infection

Special Considerations
· If urethral catheterization is traumatic, BCG should not be administered for at least 1 week
· Do not give BCG to immunosuppressed patients
· Intravesicular administration of BCG can cause conversion of a negative tuberculin skin test result to positive

Bleomycin · Blenoxane

Drug Classification
Antitumor antibiotic

Mechanism
- Produces breaks in single- and double-stranded DNA
- Cell cycle–specific acting at G_2 and M phases

Administration
- IM, IV, intraarteral, intratumoral, SC, intracavity

Therapeutic Use
- Anus
- Cervix
- Head and neck
- Hodgkin's lymphoma
- Lung
- NHL
- Penis
- Rectum
- Skin
- Testicular
- Vulva

Usual Dose and Schedule
- Single agent: 10–20 U/m^2 IV or IM once or twice a week
- Combination regimen: 30 U IV push weekly for 9–12 weeks for testicular cancer
- Intracavitary administration: 15–240 U
- Bladder instillation: 30–120 U in 30–60 ml of water instilled by urinary catheter and retained 2 hours

Side Effects/Toxicities
- Acute pulmonary edema
- Alopecia
- Desquamation
- Fever
- Headache
- Hyperpigmentation
- Lethargy
- Myelosuppression
- Nausea and vomiting
- Pain at injection site
- Pneumonitis
- Renal failure
- Stomatitis

Special Considerations
- Administer test dose (1 or 2 U) of bleomycin IM and observe for anaphylactoid, acute pulmonary, or severe hyperpyretic response
- Cumulative lifetime dose should not exceed 400 U
- Administer continuous IV infusion in a glass container

Busulfan · Myleran

Drug Classification
Alkylating agent

Mechanism
• Produces DNA-DNA cross-linking
• Produces DNA-protein cross-linking
• Activity is not cell cycle phase specific

Administration
• PO

Therapeutic Use
• CML

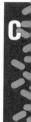

Usual Dose and Schedule

- Nonacute phase of CML: 4–12 mg/day for several weeks
- High doses with BMT: 16 mg/kg PO at 4 mg/kg/day for 4 consecutive days

Side Effects/Toxicities
• Adrenal insufficiency
• Amenorrhea
• Aplastic anemia
• Diarrhea
• Gynecomastia
• Hyperpigmentation
• Hyperuricemia
• Interstitial pulmonary fibrosis
• Leukopenia
• Ovarian suppression
• Secondary malignancies
• Thrombocytopenia

Special Considerations
• Obtain CBC weekly while patient is on therapy

Carboplatin · Paraplatin

Drug Classification
Alkylating agent

Mechanism
- Precise molecular mechanisms are unknown
- Produces DNA-DNA interstrand cross-links
- Produces DNA-protein cross-links
- Transcriptional miscoding and inhibition of DNA synthesis

Administration
- Brief IV infusions (over 15 min); continuous 24-hour IV infusion; intraperitoneal

Therapeutic Use
- Bladder
- Endometrial
- Head and neck
- Non–small cell lung
- Ovarian
- Relapsed/refractory acute leukemia
- Testicular

Usual Dose and Schedule

- Single agent: 360 mg/m^2 IV every 4 weeks
- Continuous infusion: 1000–1500 mg/m^2 over 5 days every 3 weeks; 2000 mg/m^2 over 4 days; 30 mg/m^2 day x 21 days
- Intraperitoneal: 200–650 mg/m^2 diluted in 2 L saline, instilled for 2–4 hours, then drained

Side Effects/Toxicities
- Anemia
- Diarrhea
- Hematuria
- Hepatotoxicity
- Leukopenia
- Nausea and vomiting
- Nephrotoxicity
- Thrombocytopenia

Special Considerations
- Needles and infusion sets containing aluminum should not be used

Carmustine · BCNU, BiCNU, Bis-chloro-nitrosourea

Drug Classification
Alkylating agent

Mechanism
- Inhibits a number of enzymatic reactions involved in DNA synthesis
- Produces DNA-DNA interstrand cross-links
- Produces DNA-protein cross-links
- Inhibits DNA repair

Administration
- Slow IV infusion (1–2 hours)

Therapeutic Use
- Cutaneous T-cell lymphoma
- Glioblastoma
- Hodgkin's disease
- Malignant melanoma
- Multiple myeloma

Usual Dose and Schedule

- Basic dosing schedules: 75–100 mg/m^2 IV daily for 2 consecutive days or up to 200 mg/m^2 in a single IV injection
- Autologous BMT: 450–600 mg/m^2 in a short IV infusion at a rate not greater than 3 mg/m^2/min

Side Effects/Toxicities
- Burning sensation in extremity
- Facial flushing
- Gynecomastia
- Hepatotoxicity
- Hyperpigmentation
- Leukopenia
- Nausea and vomiting
- Optic neuroretinitis
- Pain at intravenous site
- Pulmonary fibrosis
- Renal toxicity
- Thrombocytopenia

Special Considerations
- Solutions are light sensitive
- Significant absorption by plastic
- Observe for delayed myelosuppression (3–6 weeks)

Chlorambucil · Leukeran

Drug Classification
Alkylating agent

Mechanism
• Produces DNA interstrand cross-links
• Cell cycle–nonspecific

Administration
• PO

Therapeutic Use
• Breast
• Choriocarcinoma
• CLL
• Hodgkin's disease
• NHL
• Ovarian

Usual Dose and Schedule

• For CLL: 0.1–0.2 mg/kg (4–10 mg total) daily for 3–6 weeks as required for remission induction, then a maintenance schedule of 2–4 mg daily
• High dose: 108 mg/m^2 given q6h × 6

Side Effects/Toxicities
• Amenorrhea
• Azoospermia
• Coma
• Drug fever
• Hepatitis
• Lymphocytopenia
• Nausea and vomiting
• Neutropenia
• Periorbital edema
• Pulmonary fibrosis
• Secondary malignancy
• Seizures
• Skin rash
• Thrombocytopenia

Special Considerations
• Toxicity may be increased if patient has history of barbiturate use

Chlorotrianisene · Tace

Drug Classification
Hormonal agent, estrogen

Administration
• PO

Therapeutic Use
• Prostate

Mechanism
• Exact mechanism of action is unknown

Usual Dose and Schedule

• Prostate cancer: 12–15 mg/day

Side Effects/Toxicities
• Anorexia
• Areolar pigmentation
• Breast tenderness
• Feminization in males
• Gynecomastia
• Hypercalcemia
• Nausea and vomiting
• Sodium and fluid retention

Special Considerations
• Advise patient about changes in body image

Chlorozotocin · DCNU

Drug Classification
Alkylating agent

Mechanism
· Inhibits DNA and RNA synthesis
· Cell cycle–specific (S phase)

Administration
· Rapid IV injection

Therapeutic Use
· Lymphoma
· Melanoma
· Non–small cell lung cancer

Usual Dose and Schedule

• Usual dose: 5–175 mg/m^2 every 6 weeks

Side Effects/Toxicity
· Diarrhea
· Hepatotoxicity
· Local vein irritation
· Nausea and vomiting
· Nephrotoxicity
· Pulmonary fibrosis
· Stomatitis
· Thrombocytopenia

Special Considerations
· None

Cisplatin · Platinol

Drug Classification
Alkylating agent

Mechanism
- Interacts with DNA
- Produces DNA-DNA cross-links
- Produces DNA adducts and changes in DNA conformation

Administration
- IV, intraarterial, intravesical, intraperitoneal

Therapeutic Use
- Bladder
- Breast
- Colorectal
- Gastric
- Head and neck
- Non–small cell lung
- Osteosarcoma
- Ovarian
- Penile
- Pediatric brain tumors
- Small cell lung

Usual Dose and Schedule
- Typical regimens: 20 mg/m^2/day for 5 days repeated every 3 weeks; 100–120 mg/m^2 IV every 3–4 weeks; 100 mg/m^2 on days 1 and 8 repeated every 20 days
- High-dose regimen: 200 mg/m^2 per course
- Intraarterial: 120 mg/m^2 infused over 45 hours
- Intraperitoneal: 90–270 mg/m^2 in 2 L normal saline

Side Effects/Toxicities
- Anaphylaxis
- Anemia
- Atrial fibrillation
- Bundle branch block
- Cellulitis at injection site
- Hepatotoxicity
- Hypomagnesemia
- Nausea and vomiting
- Nephrotoxicity
- Ototoxicity
- Peripheral neuropathy
- SIADH
- ST- T-wave abnormalities

Special Considerations
- Should be given with great caution in patients with impaired renal function, impaired hearing, or preexisting peripheral neuropathy

C

Cladribine · 2-Chloro-2′deoxyadenosine, Leustatin

Drug Classification
Antimetabolite

Mechanism
• Leads to DNA strand breaks
• Inhibits DNA repair

Administration
• Continuous IV infusion

Therapeutic Use
• AML
• Astrocytoma
• CML
• Hairy cell leukemia
• Low-grade lymphocytic lymphoma
• NHL

Usual Dose and Schedule

• Hairy cell leukemia: 0.1 mg/kg/day × 7 days as a continuous IV infusion

Side Effects/Toxicities
• Lymphopenia
• Neutropenia
• Rash

Special Considerations
• None

Cyclophosphamide · Cytoxan, Endoxan, Neosar

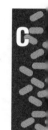

Drug Classification
Alkylating agent

Mechanism
- Forms two intracellular alkylating metabolites
- Cross-links DNA strands, preventing cell division
- Produces single-strand breaks in DNA

Administration
- PO, IV

Therapeutic Use
- Acute leukemia
- Bladder
- Breast
- Burkitt's lymphoma
- Endometrial
- Multiple myeloma
- Neuroblastoma
- Non-Hodgkin's lymphomas
- Ovarian
- Sarcoma
- Small cell lung (oat cell) cancer
- Testicular
- Wilms' tumor

Usual Dose and Schedule

- Single agent: 500–1500 mg/m^2 per treatment course, repeated every 2–4 weeks
- Continuous daily dosing: 60–120 mg/m^2 or 1–2.5 mg/kg/day
- High doses with BMT: 5.625 g/m^2 with cisplatin and carmustine; 160 mg/kg with carmustine; 1.8 g/m^2 with carmustine and etoposide; 7.2 g/m^2 with carmustine and etoposide

Side Effects/Toxicities
- Alopecia
- Amenorrhea
- Anorexia
- Bladder cancer
- Cardiotoxicity (high doses)
- Hemorrhagic cystitis
- Hepatotoxicity
- Hyponatremia
- Leukopenia
- Nausea and vomiting
- Pneumonitis
- SIADH
- Testicular atrophy
- Thrombocytopenia

Special Considerations
- Give dose in the morning, maintain ample fluid intake, and have patient empty bladder several times a day and at bedtime to decrease the likelihood of cystitis

Cytarabine · Ara-C, Cytosar-U, Cytosine arabinoside

Drug Classification
Antimetabolite

Mechanism
• Toxic metabolite acts as a competitive inhibitor of DNA polymerase
• Blocks polymerization of DNA
• S phase–specific

Administration
• SC, IM, IV push, continuous IV infusion, IT, intraperitoneal

Therapeutic Use
• AML
• ANML
• CML
• CNS leukemia
• Erythroleukemia
• Hodgkin's disease
• NHL

Usual Dose and Schedule

• Induction: 100–200 mg/m^2 IV daily as a continuous infusion for 5–7 days
• Maintenance: 100 mg/m^2 SC q12h for 4–5 days every 3–4 weeks
• Intrathecally: 40–50 mg/m^2 every 4 days in preservative-free buffered isotonic diluent
• High dose: 3.0 gm/m^2 IV over 1 hour q12h for 12 doses

Side Effects/Toxicities
• Acral erythema (palms and soles)
• Anorexia
• Cerebellar toxicity
• Diarrhea
• Flulike syndrome
• GI ulceration
• Hepatotoxicity
• Leukopenia
• Nausea and vomiting
• Pain at injection site
• Rash
• Stomatitis
• Thrombocytopenia
• Thrombophlebitis
• Urinary retention

Special Considerations
• With high doses, given in a 1-hour infusion (longer infusions enhance toxicity)

Dacarbazine · DIC, Dimethyl-triazeno-imadazole-carboxamide, DTIC-Dome

Drug Classification

Alkylating agent

Mechanism

- Exact mechanism of action is unknown
- Inhibit synthesis of protein, RNA, and DNA

Administration

- IV push, IV infusion, intraarterial, IT, intraventricular

Therapeutic Use

- Hodgkin's disease
- Malignant melanoma
- Soft tissue sarcomas

Usual Dose and Schedule

- Consecutive daily schedule: 2–4.5 mg/kg/day IV for 10 consecutive days or ≤ 250 mg/m^2 for 5 consecutive days
- Single dose: 850 mg/m^2 on day 1 of therapy with doses repeated at 3- or 4-week intervals
- High dose: 350 mg/m^2–2.5 g/m^2 given by 24-hour infusion
- Intraarterial (hepatic metastases): 200 mg/m^2/day as a 24-hour infusion in 1000 ml of D5W for 5 days or 250 mg/m^2/day for 5 consecutive days
- IT: 5–20 mg

Side Effects/Toxicities

- Alopecia
- Anemia
- Hepatotoxicity
- Extravasation
- Facial flushing
- Facial paresthesias
- Flulike syndrome
- Leukopenia
- Photosensitivity
- Nausea and vomiting
- Thrombocytopenia

Special Considerations

- Avoid extravasation
- Pain along injection site may be reduced by diluting dacarbazine in 100–200 ml of D5W and infusing over 30 minutes

Dactinomycin · Actinomycin D, Cosmegen

Drug Classification
Antitumor antibiotic

Mechanism
- Becomes noncovalently bound between purine-pyrimidine base pairs in DNA by intercalation
- Inhibits the synthesis of DNA-dependent ribosomal RNA and new messenger RNA
- Cell cycle–nonspecific

Administration
- Slow IV push, isolated arterial limb perfusion

Therapeutic Use
- Embryonal carcinoma of the testis
- Ewing's sarcoma
- Gestational choriocarcinoma
- KS
- Melanoma
- Rhabdomyosarcoma
- Testicular
- Wilms' tumor

Usual Dose and Schedule

- Children: 0.40–0.45 mg/m^2 (maximum 0.5 mg) IV daily for 5 days every 3–5 weeks
- Adults: 0.40–0.45 mg/m^2 IV on days 1–5 every 2–3 weeks; 0.5 mg IV daily for 5 days every 3–5 weeks
- Regional perfusion: 0.035 mg/kg for upper extremity; 0.05 mg/kg for lower extremity

Side Effects/Toxicities
- Acne
- Alopecia
- Anemia
- Erythema
- Hepatotoxicity
- Hyperpigmentation
- Leukopenia
- Nausea and vomiting
- Radiation "recall" skin reactions
- Thrombocytopenia

Special Considerations
- Avoid extravasation. Administer through the sidearm of a freely running IV infusion
- If given at or about the time of a chickenpox or herpes zoster infection, a severe generalized infection may occur that sometimes results in death

Daunorubicin HCl · Cerubidine, Daunomycin, Rubidomycin HCl

Drug Classification
Antitumor antibiotic

Mechanism
- Inhibits DNA and RNA synthesis
- Induces double-strand breaks in DNA by interfering with the enzyme DNA topoisomerase II

Administration
- Short IV push, short IV infusion (100 ml of D5W or normal saline over 15–30 minutes)

Therapeutic Use
- ALL
- ANLL

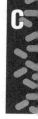

Usual Dose and Schedule

- Adult ANNL remission induction: 45–60 mg/m^2/day $\times$ 3 consecutive days
- Pediatric ALL remission induction: 25 mg/m^2 on day 1 every week
- Maximum lifetime dose: 550 mg/m^2 for adults; 300 mg/m^2 for children > 2 yr; 10 mg/kg for children < 2 yr

Side Effects/Toxicities
- Alopecia
- Congestive heart failure
- Contact dermatitis
- Extravasation
- Fever and chills
- Hepatotoxicity
- Hyperpigmentation of the nail beds
- Hyperuricemia
- Leukopenia
- Nausea and vomiting
- Nephrotoxicity
- Stomatitis
- Thrombocytopenia
- Urticaria

Special Considerations
- Does extravasate; administer over several minutes in the sidearm of a running IV infusion
- Do not administer to a patient who has a significant reduction in cardiac function (ejection fraction < 45%), angina pectoris, cardiac arrhythmias, or recent MI
- Do not exceed cumulative dose of 550 mg/m^2 (400 mg/m^2 if patient previously received radiation therapy that has included the heart)

Dexamethasone · Decadron, Dexone, Hexadrol

Drug Classification

Corticosteroid

Mechanism

· Diverse physiologic effects
· Steroid-induced inhibition of glucose transport or phosphorylation

Administration

· PO, IV

Therapeutic Use

· Antiemetic
· Relief of symptoms related to cerebral edema

Usual Dose and Schedule

· Antiemetic: 10–20 mg IV or PO for 2–4 doses in 24–48 hours
· Cerebral edema: 4–10 mg initially; 4–8 mg q6h until symptoms subside

Side Effects/Toxicities

· Cataracts
· Cushingoid syndrome
· GI bleeding
· Hyperglycemia
· Immunosuppression
· Increased ocular pressure

Special Considerations

· Acute perineal burning may occur with rapid IV administration

Diethystilbestrol Diphosphonate · DES, Stilphostrol

Drug Classification
Hormonal agent, estrogen

Mechanism
· Exact mechanism of action is unknown

Administration
· PO, IV

Therapeutic Use
· Palliative therapy for advanced breast cancer in postmenopausal female
· Palliative therapy for prostate cancer

Usual Dose and Schedule

- Breast: 1–5 mg PO t.i.d.
- Prostate: 1–3 mg/day PO

Side Effects/Toxicities
· Alteration in libido
· Areolar pigmentation
· Bone pain
· Breast tenderness
· Erythema
· Fluid retention
· Gynecomastia
· Headache
· Hyperglycemia
· Hypertension
· Nausea and vomiting
· Peripheral edema
· Sodium retention
· Thrombophlebitis

Special Considerations
· Hypercalcemia may occur with initial therapy

Doxorubicin · Adriamycin, Rubex

Drug Classification

Antitumor antibiotic

Mechanism

- Intercalates between base pairs in DNA double helix
- Inhibits the DNA repair enzyme topoisomerase II
- Acts at all phases of the cell cycle

Administration

- IV push, continuous IV infusion, intraarterial, intrapleural, topical bladder instillation

Therapeutic Use

- ALL
- AML
- Breast
- Bladder
- Ewing's sarcoma
- Hepatocellular
- Hodgkin's disease
- Neuroblastoma
- NHL
- Non–small cell lung cancer
- Ovarian
- Small cell lung cancer
- Thyroid
- Wilms' tumor

Usual Dose and Schedule

- Single dose: 60–75 mg/m^2 no more than every 3 weeks; 20 mg/m^2 once weekly; 30 mg/m^2 daily $\times$ 3 days every 4 weeks
- Intraarterial: 25 mg/m^2/day $\times$ 3 days repeated at 3 weeks, or 0.2–0.3 mg/kg for 2–20 days
- Intrapleural: 30 mg in 20 ml normal saline
- Topical bladder: 50 mg in 150 ml normal saline retained for 30 minutes

Side Effects/Toxicities

- Alopecia
- Anemia
- Congestive heart failure
- Conjunctivitis
- Extravasation
- Hyperpigmentation
- Leukopenia
- Mucositis
- Nausea and vomiting
- Phlebosclerosis
- Radiation recall
- Thrombocytopenia

Special Considerations

- Does extravasate. Administer over several minutes into the sidearm of a running IV infusion
- Do not exceed a lifetime cumulative dose of 550 mg/m^2 (450 mg/m^2 if patient previously received chest radiotherapy or is concurrently receiving cyclophosphamide)
- Do not give if patient has significantly impaired cardiac function (ejection fraction < 45%), angina pectoris, cardiac arrhythmias, or recent MI

Dromostanolone Propionate · Drolban

Drug Classification
Hormonal agent, androgen

Mechanism
· Exact mechanism of action is unknown

Administration
· IM

Therapeutic Use
· Advanced breast cancer in postmenopausal female with hormone-dependent tumor containing estrogen and/or progesterone receptors
· Protein anabolism
· Refractory anemia

Usual Dose and Schedule

· 4–7 mg/kg/week IM
· 100 mg 3 times weekly

Side Effects/Toxicities
· Alopecia
· Amenorrhea
· Anxiety
· Change in libido
· Clitoral hypertrophy
· Deepening of the voice
· Depression
· Headache
· Masculinism
· Sodium retention

Special Considerations
· Inject deep IM to minimize pain at injection site

C

Epirubicin · 4'-Epidoxorubicin, Farmorubicin, Pharmorubicin

Drug Classification
Antitumor antibiotic

Mechanism
- Intercalates into DNA to inhibit nucleic acid synthesis
- Induces protein-linked DNA double-strand breaks

Administration
- IV push, brief IV infusion (15–20 minutes), intraarterial, intraperitoneal, intravesical

Therapeutic Use
- Breast
- Chronic leukemias
- Colorectal
- Gastric
- Hepatocellular
- Malignant melanoma
- NHL
- Non–small cell lung cancer
- Ovarian
- Pancreatic
- Renal cell
- Small-cell lung cancer

Usual Dose and Schedule

- Single agent: 75–90 mg/m^2 IV every 3 weeks; 40–50 mg/m^2/day IV on 2 consecutive days every 3 weeks
- High dose: 120 mg/m^2
- Intraarterial: 20–40 mg into the hepatic artery
- Intraperitoneal: 30 mg in 60 ml normal saline
- Intravesical: 50 mg in 50 ml 0.9% sodium chloride instilled for 2 hours

Side Effects/Toxicities
- Alopecia
- Congestive heart failure
- Diarrhea
- Leukopenia
- Nausea and vomiting
- Phlebitis
- Red-orange urine
- Stomatitis
- Thrombocytopenia

Special Considerations
- Avoid extravasation
- Do not exceed a lifetime cumulative dose of 1000 mg/m^2 (use a reduced dose for patients with prior history of chest radiotherapy or treatment with anthracyclines or anthracenes)

Epoetin Alfa · Epogen, Erythropoietin, Procrit

Drug Classification
Immunoregulating agent

Mechanism
- Regulates growth of bone marrow stem cells
- Regulates proliferation, differentiation, and maturation of RBCs

Administration
- SC

Therapeutic Use
- Anemia associated with CTX, CRF, or AZT therapy

Usual Dose and Schedule
- Starting dose: 150 U/kg SC

Side Effects/Toxicities
- Diarrhea
- Hypertension
- Rash
- Seizures
- Thrombotic events

Special Considerations
- Do not shake vial during preparation

Estradiol (Estrace)

Drug Classification
Hormonal agent, estrogen

Mechanism
• Exact mechanism of action is unknown

Administration
• PO

Therapeutic Use
• Breast cancer in males and postmenopausal females
• Prostate

Usual Dose and Schedule

- • Breast: 10 mg t.i.d.
- • Prostate: 1–2 mg t.i.d.

Side Effects/Toxicities
• Alteration in libido
• Areolar pigmentation
• Bone pain
• Breast tenderness
• Erythema
• Fluid retention
• Gynecomastia
• Headache
• Hyperglycemia
• Hypertension
• Nausea and vomiting
• Peripheral edema
• Sodium retention
• Thrombophlebitis

Special Considerations
• Hypercalcemia may occur with initial therapy

Estradiol Valerate · Delestrogen, Estravel

Drug Classification
Hormonal agent, estrogen

Mechanism
· Exact mechanism of action is unknown

Administration
· IM

Therapeutic Use
· Breast cancer in males and estrogen receptor–positive tumors in females
· Prostate

Usual Dose and Schedule

· At least 30 mg IM every 1–2 weeks

Side Effects/Toxicities
· Alteration in libido
· Areolar pigmentation
· Bone pain
· Breast tenderness
· Erythema
· Fluid retention
· Gynecomastia
· Headache
· Hyperglycemia
· Hypertension
· Nausea and vomiting
· Peripheral edema
· Sodium retention
· Thrombophlebitis

Special Considerations
· Hypercalcemia may occur with initial therapy

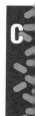

Estramustine Phosphate · Emcyt, Estracyte

Drug Classification
Chemical combination of estradiol phosphate and nitrogen mustard

Mechanism
- Estrogenic portion of the molecule may act as a carrier to facilitate selective uptake of the drug into cells with estradiol hormone receptors
- Binds to microtubules to promote disassembly
- Works at any phase in the cell cycle

Administration
- PO, IV push

Therapeutic Use
- Metastatic prostate cancer

Usual Dose and Schedule
- PO: 140–1400 mg/day; 20–25 mg/kg/day
- IV: 300 mg/day

Side Effects/Toxicities
- Gynecomastia
- Hepatotoxicity
- Nausea and vomiting
- Rash
- Thrombocytopenia
- Thrombophlebitis (IV use)

Special Considerations
- Should not be administered to patients with thrombophlebitis or thromboembolic disorders
- Contraindications: peptic ulceration, severe liver disease, cardiac disease

Estrogen Conjugate · Premarin

Drug Classification
Hormonal agent, estrogen

Mechanism
· Exact mechanism of action is unknown

Administration
· PO, IV

Therapeutic Use
· Breast cancer in males and postmenopausal females
· Prostate cancer

Usual Dose and Schedule

· Breast: 10 mg PO t.i.d.
· Prostate: 1.25–2.5 mg PO t.i.d.

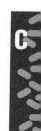

Side Effects/Toxicities
· Alteration in libido
· Areolar pigmentation
· Bone pain
· Breast tenderness
· Erythema
· Fluid retention
· Gynecomastia
· Headache
· Hyperglycemia
· Hypertension
· Nausea and vomiting
· Peripheral edema
· Sodium retention
· Thrombophlebitis

Special Considerations
· Hypercalcemia may occur with initial therapy

Estrogen, Esterified · Estratab, Menest

Drug Classification
Hormonal agent, estrogen

Mechanism
· Exact mechanism of action is unknown

Administration
· PO

Therapeutic Use
· Breast cancer in males and postmenopausal females
· Prostate cancer

Usual Dose and Schedule

· Breast: 10 mg PO t.i.d.
· Prostate: 1.25–2.5 mg PO t.i.d.

Side Effects/Toxicities
· Alteration in libido
· Areolar pigmentation
· Bone pain
· Breast tenderness
· Erythema
· Fluid retention
· Gynecomastia
· Headache
· Hyperglycemia
· Hypertension
· Nausea and vomiting
· Peripheral edema
· Sodium retention
· Thrombophlebitis

Special Considerations
· Hypercalcemia may occur with initial therapy

Ethinyl Estradiol · Estinyl

Drug Classification
Hormonal agent, estrogen

Mechanism
· Exact mechanism of action is unknown

Administration
· PO

Therapeutic Use
· Breast cancer in males and estrogen receptor–positive tumors in females
· Prostate cancer

Usual Dose and Schedule

- Breast: 1 mg PO t.i.d.
- Prostate: 0.5–1 mg PO t.i.d.

Side Effects/Toxicities
· Alteration in libido
· Areolar pigmentation
· Bone pain
· Breast tenderness
· Erythema
· Fluid retention
· Gynecomastia
· Headache
· Hyperglycemia
· Hypertension
· Nausea and vomiting
· Peripheral edema
· Sodium retention
· Thrombophlebitis

Special Considerations
· Hypercalcemia may occur with initial therapy

C

Etoposide · Epipodophyllotoxin, VePesid, VP-16

Drug Classification

Mitotic inhibitor

Mechanism

- Produces protein-linked DNA strand breaks by inhibiting DNA topoisomerase II activity
- Maximal effects occur in G_2

Administration

- PO, IV infusion, intrapleural, intraperitoneal

Therapeutic Use

- ALL
- Diffuse histiocytic lymphoma
- Hodgkin's disease
- Lymphosarcoma
- Reticulum cell sarcoma
- Small cell bronchogenic carcinoma
- Small cell (oat cell) lung
- Testicular

Usual Dose and Schedule

- Lung: 35 mg/m^2 IV $\times$ 4 days to 50 mg/m^2 $\times$ 5 days, every 3–4 weeks
- Testicular: 50–100 mg/m^2 IV on days 1 through 5 or 100 mg/m^2 on days 1, 3, and 5, every 3–4 weeks
- Oral: administer twice the IV dose rounded to the nearest 50 mg
- High dose: 500 mg/500 ml of saline administered over 1 hour $\times$ 4 doses

Side Effects/Toxicities

- Allergic reactions
- Alopecia
- Anorexia
- Bronchospasm
- Chemical phlebitis
- Fatigue
- Fever
- Headache
- Hypotension
- Leukopenia
- Nausea and vomiting
- Somnolence
- Stomatitis
- Thrombocytopenia

Special Considerations

- Administer as a 30–60 minute infusion to avoid severe hypotension
- Avoid extravasation
- All solutions should be examined for fine precipitates and mixed immediately prior to use

Filgrastim · Granulocyte colony–stimulating factor [G-CSF], Neupogen

Drug Classification
Immunoregulating agent

Mechanism
- Promotes proliferation and differentiation of neutrophils
- Enhances functional properties of mature neutrophils

Administration
- SC, IV

Therapeutic Use
- Decreases the incidence of infection in neutropenic patients

Usual Dose and Schedule

- 5 μg/kg/day administered as a single daily dose for up to 2 weeks

Side Effects/Toxicities
- Bone pain

Special Considerations
- Human G-CSF should not be given to patients with a history of known sensitivity to *E. coli*–derived proteins

Floxuridine · FUDR

Drug Classification

Antimetabolite

Mechanism

- Preactivated form of 5-FU
- Active metabolite binds to and inhibits thymidylate synthetase in concert with reduced folate cofactors
- S phase–specific
- Inhibits DNA synthesis

Administration

- IV, intraarterial, intraventricular, intracavitary

Therapeutic Use

- Biliary tract
- Colon
- GI tract adenocarcinoma
- Liver
- Oral cavity

Usual Dose and Schedule

- Intraarterial: 0.1–0.6 mg/kg/day for 1–6 weeks; 0.4–0.6 mg/kg/day $\times$ 14 days (for intrahepatic administration)
- IV continuous infusion: 0.5–1.0 mg/kg/day for 6–15 days (induction); 15 mg/kg every other day until relapse (maintenance)
- Intraventricular: 4–16 mg
- Intracavitary: 30 mg/kg (intrapleural or intraperitoneal)

Side Effects/Toxicities

- Abdominal cramps
- Abdominal pain
- Alopecia
- Anemia
- Anorexia
- Biliary cirrhosis
- Blurred vision
- Depression
- Diarrhea
- Edema
- Gastric ulceration
- Hepatotoxicity
- Hyperpigmentation of veins
- Lethargy
- Leukopenia
- Mucositis
- Nausea and vomiting
- Nystagmus
- Pruritus
- Rash
- Thrombocytopenia
- Vertigo

Special Considerations

- Abdominal pain and/or GI symptoms are indications to discontinue intraarterial therapy because hemorrhage or perforation may occur
- GI toxicity may be reduced by delivering continuous infusions between 3:00 PM and 9:00 PM

Fludarabine Phosphate · Fludara, 2-Fluoro-Ara-AMP

Drug Classification
Antimetabolite

Mechanism
- Inhibits DNA synthesis by inhibition of ribonucleotide reductase and DNA polymerase

Administration
- Short IV infusion, rapid loading dose/continuous IV infusion, intraperitoneal (investigational)

Therapeutic Use
- ALL
- ANLL
- CLL
- Gliomas
- Low-grade lymphomas
- Mycosis fungoides

Usual Dose and Schedule

- Short infusion: 18–30 mg/m^2/day $\times$ 5 as a 30-minute infusion
- Loading dose: 20 mg/m^2 (rapid IV infusion) followed by 30 mg/m^2/day by continuous infusion for 48 hours
- Intraperitoneal: 4–25 mg/m^2 every 28 days

Side Effects/Toxicities
- Anemia
- CNS toxicity
- Diarrhea
- Granulocytopenia
- Interstitial pneumonitis
- Lymphocytopenia
- Nausea and vomiting
- Skin rash
- Somnolence
- Thrombocytopenia
- Tumor lysis syndrome

Special Considerations
- Patients with preexisting neurologic disease should be treated cautiously to avoid serious CNS complications
- Allopurinol should be administered prophylactically to avoid tumor lysis syndrome in patients with CLL
- Cumulative myelosuppression can occur

C

5-Fluorouracil · Adrucil, Efudex, 5-FU

Drug Classification

Antimetabolite

Mechanism

- Acts as a "false" pyrimidine to inhibit the formation of thymidine
- S phase–specific

Administration

- IV push, continuous IV infusion, PO, topical, intraarterial, portal vein infusion, intraperitoneal, intracavitary

Therapeutic Use

- Basal cell
- Bladder
- Breast
- Colon
- Head and neck
- Pancreas
- Prostate
- Rectal
- Renal cell
- Squamous cell of the esophagus
- Stomach

Usual Dose and Schedule

- Conventional bolus dose: 400–500 mg/m^2 daily $\times$ 4 days as a bolus or an infusion
- Maintenance dose: 200–250 mg/m^2 every other day for 4 days, repeated in 4 weeks; 500–600 mg/m^2 IV weekly as a continuous infusion or bolus
- Intraarterial: 20–30 mg/kg/day $\times$ 4, then 15 mg/kg/day $\times$ 17 days (hepatic); 12–15 mg/kg/day $\times$ 4–5 days (biliary tract)

Side Effects/Toxicities

- Acute cerebellar syndrome
- Alopecia
- Diarrhea
- Esophagitis
- Headache
- Hyperpigmentation of the nail beds
- Leukopenia
- Maculopapular rash
- MI
- Nausea and vomiting
- Palmar-plantar erythrodysesthesias
- Photosensitivity
- Visual disturbances
- Proctitis
- Stomatitis
- Thrombocytopenia

Special Considerations

- 5-FU (even topical) should never be given during pregnancy
- Patients who have had an adrenalectomy may require increased doses of cortisone

Fluoxymesterone · Halotestin

Drug Classification
Hormonal agent, androgen

Mechanism
· Exact mechanism of action is unknown

Administration
· PO

Therapeutic Use
· Advanced breast cancer

Usual Dose and Schedule
· 10–30 mg/day

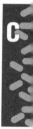

Side Effects/Toxicities
· Alopecia
· Amenorrhea
· Anxiety
· Change in libido
· Clitoral hypertrophy
· Deepening of the voice
· Depression
· Headache
· Masculinism
· Sodium retention

Special Considerations
· Hypercalcemia may occur with initial therapy

Flutamide · Eulexin

Drug Classification
Hormonal agent, androgen receptor antagonist

Mechanism
- Inhibits the uptake and binding of the androgens testosterone and dihydrotestosterone to specific receptors in hormonally dependent prostate cells

Administration
- PO

Therapeutic Use
- Advanced prostate cancer

Usual Dose and Schedule
- 250 mg t.i.d.

Side Effects/Toxicities
- Anorexia
- Diarrhea
- Edema
- Gynecomastia
- Hot flashes
- Hypertension
- Impotence
- Loss of libido
- Nausea and vomiting
- Photosensitivity

Special Considerations
- None

Gallium Nitrate · Ganite

Drug Classification
Miscellaneous agent

Mechanism
· Inhibits bone resorption of calcium

Administration
· IV infusion

Therapeutic Use
· Treatment of cancer-related hypercalcemia

Usual Dose and Schedule

· 200 mg/m^2/day $\times$ 5 days

Side Effects/Toxicities
· Hypocalcemia
· Hypophosphatemia
· Hypotension
· Nephrotoxicity
· Optic neuropathy

Special Considerations
· Should not be given to patients with a serum creatinine > 2.5 mg/dl
· Provide adequate hydration prior to administration

C

Goserelin Acetate · Zoladex

Drug Classification
Hormonal agent, inhibitor of gonadotropin release from the pituitary

Mechanism
- Superpotent agonist of LH-RH
- Continuous stimulation produced by goserelin leads to near complete inhibition of FSH and LH release
- Testosterone, progesterone, and estradiol are reduced to castrate levels

Administration
- SC injection into abdominal body fat

Therapeutic Use
- Advanced prostate cancer
- Premenopausal women with hormonally dependent breast cancer

Usual Dose and Schedule
- Adult dose: 3.6 mg every 28 days

Side Effects/Toxicities
- Anorexia
- Bone pain
- Decreased libido
- Dizziness
- Edema
- Gynecomastia
- Hot flashes
- Lethargy
- Nausea
- Rash at the injection site
- Sweating

Special Considerations
- Local anesthetic may be given prior to injection

Hydrocortisone Sodium Succinate · Hydrocortone

Drug Classification
Corticosteroid

Mechanism
• Diverse physiologic effects
• Steroid-induced inhibition of glucose
  transport or phosphorylation

Administration
• PO, IM, IV

Therapeutic Use
• Postadrenalectomy

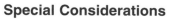

Usual Dose and Schedule

• 25–30 mg/day

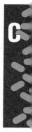

Side Effects/Toxicities
• Cataracts
• Cushingoid syndrome
• GI bleeding
• Hyperglycemia
• Immunosuppression
• Increased ocular pressure

Special Considerations
• None

Hydroxyprogesterone · Prodrox (Legere) 250

Drug Classification
Hormonal agent, progestin

Mechanism
• Exact biochemical action is unknown
• Oxidizes estradiol to a less potent form

Administration
• IM

Therapeutic Use
• Breast
• Endometrial
• Well-differentiated renal cell

Usual Dose and Schedule

• 2–5 g IM weekly to remission; then 1 g IM weekly maintenance

Side Effects/Toxicities
• Alopecia
• Backache
• Birth defects
• Cramps
• Dyspnea
• Gluteal abscess
• Hypercalcemia
• Nausea and vomiting
• Vaginal bleeding

Special Considerations
• Some patients may be sensitive to the oil carrier

Hydroxyurea · Hydrea, Hydroxycarbamide, Litalir

Drug Classification
Other

Mechanism
· Blocks the ribonucleotide reductase system in cells
· Inhibits DNA synthesis

Administration
· PO, IV (investigational)

Therapeutic Use
· CML
· Head and neck
· Malignant melanoma
· Refractory ovarian

Usual Dose and Schedule

· CML: 50–75 mg/kg IV when the WBC count is > 100,000/mm^3. With lower initial blast counts, daily oral dose of 10–20 mg/kg
· Solid tumors: 80 mg/kg as a single dose every third day or 20–30 mg/kg/day

Side Effects/Toxicities
· Acral erythema
· Anemia
· Constipation
· Convulsions
· Diarrhea
· Dizziness
· Dysuria
· Facial erythema
· Fever
· Hallucinations
· Headache
· Leukopenia
· Maculopapular rash
· Nausea and vomiting
· Radiation "recall"
· Stomatitis
· Thrombocytopenia

Special Considerations
· Daily dose must be adjusted for blood counts

C

Idarubicin HCl · 4-Demethoxy-Daunorubicin, Idamycin

Drug Classification
Antitumor antibiotic

Mechanism
• Produces lesions in DNA
• Inhibition of DNA and RNA synthesis

Administration
• IV brief infusion (10–15 min), PO (investigational)

Therapeutic Use
• ALL
• ANLL
• CML

Usual Dose and Schedule

• Remission induction in ANLL: 12 mg/m^2/day for 3 consecutive days

Side Effects/Toxicities
• Alopecia
• Cardiotoxicity
• Diarrhea
• Extravasation
• Hepatotoxicity
• Leukopenia
• Mucositis
• Nausea and vomiting
• Rash
• Thrombocytopenia
• Uticaria

Special Considerations
• Cardiac toxicity may be less than with daunorubicin; maximum dose not yet established

Ifosfamide · Holoxan, Ifex

Drug Classification
Alkylating agent

Mechanism
- Cross-links DNA strands
- Cell cycle–nonspecific

Administration
- IV

Therapeutic Use
- Acute leukemia
- Breast
- Bronchogenic carcinoma
- Chronic leukemia
- Germ-cell testicular
- Hodgkin's disease
- Non–small cell lung
- Ovarian
- Soft tissue sarcoma

Usual Dose and Schedule
- Testicular: 1.2 g/m^2/day for 5 consecutive days
- Single agent: 2400 mg/m^2/day IV push for 3 consecutive days
- Continuous infusion: 4 g/m^2 as a 24-hour slow infusion repeated every 3 weeks

Side Effects/Toxicities
- Alopecia
- Ataxia
- Confusion
- Dysuria
- Hemorrhagic cystitis
- Hepatotoxicity
- Lethargy
- Leukopenia
- Nausea and vomiting
- Nephrotoxicity
- Seizures
- Sterile phlebitis
- Stupor
- Urinary frequency
- Weakness

Special Considerations
- Patient must be well hydrated
- Mesna, given IV or PO, is required to prevent hemorrhagic cystitis
- Previous radiation and/or chemotherapy may necessitate dosage adjustments

Immune Globulin · Gamastan, Gamimune N, Gammagard, Gammar, Gammar-IV, IG IV, Iveegam, Sandoglobulin, Venoglobulin-I

Drug Classification

Immunomodulating agent

Mechanism

- Provides passive immunity against many infections

Administration

- IM, IV

Therapeutic Use

- Prevention of bacterial infections in patients with B-cell CLL
- Idiopathic thrombocytopenia purpura

Usual Dose and Schedule

- Immunodeficiency: 200–400 mg/kg/month
- Idiopathic thrombocytopenia purpura: 400 mg/kg/day for 2–5 days or 1 g/kg/day for 1–2 days

Side Effects/Toxicities

- Back pain
- Chest pain
- Cyanosis
- Diuresis
- Dyspnea
- Faintness
- Headache
- Hip pain
- Light-headedness
- Malaise
- Nausea
- Nephrotic syndrome
- Pain at injection site (IM)
- Urticaria
- Wheezing

Special Considerations

- IM form should be used cautiously in patients with thrombocytopenia
- Anaphylactic reactions have been reported
- Bring powder and diluent to room temperature prior to reconstitution. Do not shake the vial.

Interferon Alfa-2a · INF-A, Intron A, Roferon-A

Drug Classification
Immunoregulating agent

Mechanism
- Direct inhibition of tumor cell growth
- Modulation of host immune response
- Activation of natural killer cells
- Modulation of antibody production
- Induction of major histocompatibility antigens

Administration
- IM, SC, intraperitoneal, intralesional

Therapeutic Use
- AIDS-related Kaposi's sarcoma
- CML
- Cutaneous T-cell lymphoma
- Hairy cell leukemia
- Malignant melanoma
- Mycosis fungoides
- NHL
- Renal cell carcinoma

Usual Dose and Schedule
- Hairy cell leukemia: for induction, 3 million IU daily × 16–24 weeks; for maintenance, 3 million IU 3 times weekly for up to 24 months
- Kaposi's sarcoma: for induction, 36 million IU/day for 10–12 weeks; for maintenance, 36 million IU 3 times per week

Side Effects/Toxicities
- Alopecia
- Anemia
- Anorexia
- Decreased attention span
- Decreased short-term memory
- Dry skin
- Elevated liver function tests
- Flulike syndrome
- Insomnia
- Leg cramps
- Myelosuppression
- Nausea and vomiting
- Neutropenia
- Paranoia
- Paresthesias
- Poor concentration
- Pruritus
- Psychoses
- Taste alterations
- Weight loss
- Xerostomia

Special Considerations
- Evaluate patient's hydration status prior to drug administration to prevent dehydration
- Use drug cautiously in patients with a history of cardiovascular or pulmonary disease or diabetes mellitus

Interferon Alfa-2b

Drug Classification
Immunoregulating agent

Mechanism
- Modulates the immune response
- Has an antiproliferative effect on tumor cells

Administration
- IM, SC, intralesional

Therapeutic Use
- AIDS-associated Kaposi's sarcoma
- Chronic hepatitis (non-A, non-B/C, and B)
- Hairy cell leukemia

Usual Dose and Schedule

- Hairy cell leukemia: 2 million IU/m^2, 3 times a week
- KS: 30 million IU/m^2, 3 times a week

Side Effect/Toxicities
- Abdominal fullness
- Altered taste
- Anemia
- Anorexia
- Bronchospasm
- Chills
- Conjunctivitis
- Decreased mental status
- Depression
- Diarrhea
- Dry mouth
- Fatigue
- Fever
- Flulike syndrome
- Hypotension
- Impotence
- Leukopenia
- Myalgia
- Nausea
- Pruritus
- Rash
- Seizures
- Sleep disturbances
- Thrombocytopenia
- Vomiting
- Weight loss

Special Considerations
- Hypersensitivity reactions can occur
- Use cautiously in patients with severe cardiovascular, renal, or hepatic disease
- Use cautiously in patients who have received radiation therapy

Interleukin-1 (lymphocyte-activating factor [LAF]; endogenous pyrogen)

Drug Classification
Immunoregulating agent

Mechanism
- Exhibits some direct antiproliferative effects
- Stimulates growth factor production
- Augments T-cell cytotoxicity
- Augments B-cell activation
- Mediates the inflammatory proteins

Administration
- IV

Therapeutic Use
- Malignant melanoma
- Ovarian

Usual Dose and Schedule
- 0.1 µg/kg/day for 7 days; repeated at 2-week intervals

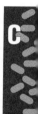

Side Effects/Toxicities
- Arthralgias
- Fever
- Headache
- Hypotension
- Myalgias
- Nausea and vomiting
- Phlebitis
- Pulmonary infiltrates
- Rigors
- Weight gain

Special Considerations
- Must be diluted with human serum albumin after initial reconstitution

Leucovorin Calcium · Calcium Folinate, Wellcovorin

Drug Classification
Reduced derivative of folic acid

Mechanism
- Competes effectively with methotrexate for transport into mammalian cells
- Used to circumvent the effects of high-dose methotrexate

Administration
- PO, IV push, IV continuous, IM

Therapeutic Use
- Modulates the effect of 5-FU
- Nutritional supplement
- "Rescue" after high-dose methotrexate

Usual Dose and Schedule

- Osteogenic sarcoma: 6–15 mg q6h $\times$ 12
- Epidermoid tumors: 40 mg/m^2 over 6 hours, then 25 mg q6h for 4 doses
- Solid tumors: 10 mg/m^2 q6h $\times$ 12

Side Effects/Toxicities
- Allergic sensitization

Special Considerations
- Progressive accumulation of the metabolite of L-leucovorin can occur in the CSF and decrease the antitumor activity of methotrexate against meningeal leukemia

Leuprolide Acetate · Leuprorelin Acetate, Lupron

Drug Classification

Hormonal agent, superpotent gonadotropin-releasing hormone agonist

Mechanism

- Binds to cell surface receptors in the pituitary
- Causes the release of FSH and LH
- Continual agonist activity of leuprolide at the pituitary chronically suppresses FSH and LH release

Administration

- SC, IM

Therapeutic Use

- Advanced prostate cancer
- Metastatic breast
- Refractory ovarian

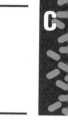

Usual Dose and Schedule

- 1 mg/day by SC injection
- 7.5 mg IM as a monthly injection

Side Effects/Toxicities

- Dysuria
- Gynecomastia
- Hot flashes
- Paresthesias
- Peripheral edema
- Weakness

Special Considerations

- None

Levamisole · Ergamisol

Drug Classification
Immunorestorative agent

Mechanism
- Mediates IL-2-induced T-lymphocyte proliferation
- Restores macrophage and T-lymphocyte function

Administration
- PO

Therapeutic Use
- Duke's C carcinoma of the colon with 5-FU

Usual Dose and Schedule

- Initial therapy: 50 mg q8hr for 3 days
- Maintenance dose: 50 mg q8hr for 3 days every 2 weeks × 1 year in combination with 5-FU

Side Effects/Toxicities
- Abdominal pain
- Anorexia
- Arthralgias
- Blurred vision
- Constipation
- Diarrhea
- Dizziness
- Fatigue
- Fever
- Headache
- Myelosuppression
- Nausea and vomiting
- Somnolence
- Stomatitis
- Taste alterations

Special Considerations
- May produce "Antabuse-like" side effects when given concomitantly with alcohol. Instruct patient to abstain from alcohol.

Lomustine · CCNU, CeeNu

Drug Classification
Alkylating agent

Mechanism
- Produces DNA-DNA cross-links
- Produces DNA-protein cross-links
- Cell cycle–nonspecific

Administration
- PO

Therapeutic Use
- Brain tumors
- Gastric cancer
- Hodgkin's disease
- Multiple myeloma
- Non–small cell lung
- Prostate cancer

Usual Dose and Schedule
- Single agent: 100–300 mg/m^2
- Combination: 30–75 mg/m^2

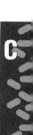

Side Effects/Toxicities
- Alopecia
- Anorexia
- Ataxia
- Confusion
- Diarrhea
- Hepatotoxicity
- Lethargy
- Leukopenia
- Nausea and vomiting
- Nephrotoxicity
- Stomatitis
- Thrombocytopenia

Special Considerations
- Delayed myelosuppression can occur

Mechlorethamine HCl · Mustargen, Nitrogen Mustard

Drug Classification
Alkylating agent

Mechanism
- Inhibits DNA synthesis
- Inhibits protein synthesis

Administration
- IV push, intracavity, topical, intralesional

Therapeutic Use
- Hodgkin's disease
- NHL

Usual Dose and Schedule

- Single dose: 0.4 mg/kg $\times$ 4 doses
- MOPP regimen: 6.0 mg/m^2 on days 1 and 8 of a 14-day cycle
- Intracavitary: 0.2–0.4 mg/kg

Side Effects/Toxicities
- Amenorrhea
- Drowsiness
- Fever
- Granulocytopenia
- Hyperpyrexia
- Nausea and vomiting
- Maculopapular rash
- Thrombocytopenia
- Thrombophlebitis
- Thrombosis
- Weakness

Special Considerations
- Avoid extravasation
- Use within 15–30 minutes of preparation

Medroxyprogesterone · Provera

Drug Classification
Hormonal agent, progestin

Mechanism
· Exact biochemical action is unknown
· Oxidizes estradiol to a less potent form

Administration
· PO, IM

Therapeutic Use
· Breast
· Endometrial
· Renal cell

Usual Dose and Schedule
· Initial dose: 400–1000 mg/week
· Later dose: 400 mg/month

Side Effects/Toxicities
· Amenorrhea
· Breast tenderness
· Cholestatic jaundice
· Edema
· Headache
· Insomnia
· Nausea and vomiting
· Nervousness
· Pain at injection site
· Pruritus
· Somnolence
· Thrombophlebitis
· Urticaria
· Vaginal bleeding

Special Considerations
· Administer deep IM
· Shake vial vigorously

Megestrol Acetate · Megace

Drug Classification
Hormonal agent, progestin

Mechanism
- Exact biochemical action is unknown
- Oxidizes estradiol to a less potent agent

Administration
- PO

Therapeutic Use
- Breast
- Endometrial
- Renal cell

Usual Dose and Schedule

- Breast: 40 mg q.i.d.
- Endometrial: 40–320 mg/day in divided doses

Side Effects/Toxicities
- Alopecia
- Amenorrhea
- Breast tenderness
- Carpal tunnel syndrome
- Cholestatic jaundice
- Edema
- Headache
- Insomnia
- Nausea and vomiting
- Nervousness
- Pruritus
- Somnolence
- Thrombophlebitis
- Urticaria
- Vaginal bleeding

Special Considerations
- None

Melphalan · Alkeran, L-PAM, L-Phenylalanine Mustard

Drug Classification
Alkylating agent

Mechanism
- Forms DNA cross-links
- Cell cycle–nonspecific

Administration
- PO, slow IV infusion, intraarterial, intraperitoneal

Therapeutic Use
- Breast
- Multiple myeloma
- Ovarian
- Rhabdomyosarcoma
- Sarcomas
- Testicular

Usual Dose and Schedule

- Breast: 0.15 mg/kg/day for 5 days
- Multiple myeloma: 9 mg/m^2 or 0.25 mg/kg/day for 4–7 days
- Ovarian: 1 mg/kg IV over 8 hours, every 4 weeks
- Regional: axillary, 0.75 mg/kg; femoral, 1.2 mg/kg

Side Effects/Toxicities
- Alopecia
- Dermatitis
- Hypersensitivity reactions
- Leukopenia
- Pulmonary fibrosis
- Stomatitis
- Thrombocytopenia

Special Considerations
- Myelosuppression may be delayed

Mercaptopurine · 6-MP, Purinethol

Drug Classification
Antimetabolite

Mechanism
• Inhibits RNA synthesis
• S phase–specific

Administration
• PO, IV push, continuous IV infusion

Therapeutic Use
• ALL
• CML
• NHL

Usual Dose and Schedule

• Oral: 80–100 mg/m^2/day or 2.5 mg/kg/day
• IV infusion: 50 mg/m^2/hour for no longer than 48 hours

Side Effects/Toxicities
• Anemia
• Anorexia
• Drug fever
• Dry, scaling rash
• Eosinophilia
• Hematuria
• Hepatotoxicity
• Leukopenia
• Mucositis
• Nausea and vomiting
• Thrombocytopenia

Special Considerations
• Decrease dose by 75% when used concurrently with allopurinol

Mesna · Mesnex, Uromitexan

Drug Classification
Selective urinary tract protectant

Mechanism
- Binds to the toxic metabolite acrolein in urine
- Selective for the urinary tract

Administration
- PO, IV

Therapeutic Use
- Urinary tract protectant for oxazophosphorine-type alkylating agents

Usual Dose and Schedule

- IV mesna: typically given in 3 divided doses, each at 20% of the ifosfamide or cyclophosphamide dose on a mg/kg basis

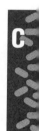

Side Effects/Toxicities
- Allergy
- Bad taste
- Diarrhea
- Fatigue
- Headache
- Hypotension
- Limb pain
- Nausea

Special Considerations
- First dose administered 15 minutes before the oxazophosphorine; then a dose is administered 4 and 8 hours later
- Oral mesna has a disagreeable sulfur odor and should be diluted (1:1 or 1:10) in carbonated cola or fruit juice

Methotrexate · Folex, Mexate, MTX

Drug Classification
Antimetabolite

Mechanism
- Inhibits purine synthesis
- Inhibits DNA, RNA, and protein synthesis
- S phase–specific

Administration
- PO, IM, IV, intraarterial, IT

Therapeutic Use
- ALL
- AML
- Breast
- Burkitt's lymphoma
- Chorioadenoma
- Choriocarcinoma
- Chorioepithelioma
- Epidermoid cancer of the head and neck
- Hydatidiform mole
- Lung
- NHL
- Osteogenic sarcoma
- Ovarian

Usual Dose and Schedule

- Conventional dose: 15–20 mg/m^2 PO, twice a week; 30–50 mg/m^2 PO or IM, weekly; 15 mg/m^2 × 5 days IV or IM, every 2–3 weeks
- Intermediate dose: 50–150 mg/m^2 IV push, every 2–3 weeks; 240 mg/m^2 IV infusion, every 4–7 days; 0.5–1 g/m^2 IV infusion (36–48 hours), every 2–3 weeks
- High dose: 1–12 g/m^2 IV (1–24 hours), every 1–3 weeks

Side Effects/Toxicities
- Alopecia
- Anemia
- Anorexia
- Blurred vision
- Depigmentation
- Diarrhea
- Dizziness
- Erythematous rashes
- Folliculitis
- Gingivitis
- Glossitis
- Hepatotoxicity
- Hyperpigmentation
- Leukopenia
- Malaise
- Nausea and vomiting
- Nephrotoxicity
- Pharyngitis
- Photosensitivity
- Pruritus
- Stomatitis
- Thrombocytopenia
- Ulcerative stomatitis
- Urticaria
- Vasculitis

Special Considerations
- High-dose methotrexate (> 80 mg/m^2) requires measurement of serum methotrexate levels
- Intrathecal methotrexate must be mixed in buffered physiologic solution without preservatives
- Oral anticoagulants may be potentiated by methotrexate

Methylprednisolone · Medrol

Drug Classification
Corticosteroid

Mechanism
- Diverse physiologic effects
- Steroid-induced inhibition of glucose transport or phosphorylation

Administration
- Oral

Therapeutic Use
- Leukemia
- Lymphoma
- Mycosis fungoides

Usual Dose and Schedule
- Dose varies with type and severity of disease

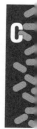

Side Effects/Toxicities
- Cataracts
- Cushingoid syndrome
- GI bleeding
- Hyperglycemia
- Immunosuppression
- Increased ocular pressure

Special Considerations
- None

Methylprednisolone Sodium Succinate · Solu-Medrol

Drug Classification
Corticosteroid

Mechanism
• Diverse physiologic effects
• Steroid-induced inhibition of glucose
  transport or phosphorylation

Administration
• IM, IV

Therapeutic Use
• Leukemia
• Lymphoma
• Mycosis fungoides

Usual Dose and Schedule

• Dose varies with type and severity of disease

Side Effects/Toxicities
• Cataracts
• Cushingoid syndrome
• GI bleeding
• Hyperglycemia
• Immunosuppression
• Increased ocular pressure

Special Considerations
• Acute perineal burning may occur with rapid IV administration

Methyltestosterone · Oreton Methyl

Drug Classification
Hormonal agent, androgen

Mechanism
• Exact mechanism of action is unknown

Administration
• PO, buccal

Therapeutic Use
• Breast
• Protein anabolism

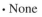

Usual Dose and Schedule

• Oral: 50–200 mg/day
• Buccal: 25–100 mg/day for 4 weeks

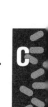

Side Effects/Toxicities
• Alopecia
• Amenorrhea
• Anxiety
• Change in libido
• Clitoral hypertrophy
• Deepening of the voice
• Depression
• Headache
• Masculinism
• Sodium retention

Special Considerations
• None

Mitomycin C · Mutamycin

Drug Classification
Antitumor antibiotic

Mechanism
- Cross-links complementary DNA strands
- Inhibits DNA synthesis
- Cell cycle–nonspecific

Administration
- IV, intravesicular, continuous IV infusion

Therapeutic Use
- Bladder
- Breast
- Cervical
- CML
- Colon
- Gallbladder
- Gastric
- Head and neck
- Non–small cell lung
- Ovarian
- Pancreas
- Uterine

Usual Dose and Schedule

- Single agent: 20 mg/m^2 IV every 6–8 weeks
- Combination regimen: 10 mg/m^2 every 6–8 weeks
- Intravesicular: 20 mg/20 ml in distilled water, retain 3 hours

Side Effects/Toxicities
- Alopecia
- Anemia
- Anorexia
- Confusion
- Drowsiness
- Extravasation
- Fatigue
- Interstitial pneumonia
- Leukopenia
- Nausea and vomiting
- Nephrotoxicity
- Purple-colored nail beds
- Stomatitis
- Thrombocytopenia
- Venoocclusive disease of the liver

Special Considerations
- Administer slow IV push through the sideport of a freely running IV line

Mitotane · Lysodren

Drug Classification
Miscellaneous agent

Mechanism
· Suppresses adrenal steroid production
· Modifies peripheral steroid metabolism
· Cytotoxic to adrenal cortical cells

Administration
· PO

Therapeutic Use
· Adrenal cortical carcinoma

Usual Dose and Schedule

· Begin with 2–6 g daily in 3–4 divided doses and build to a maximum tolerated daily dose (usually 8–10 g, although it may range from 2–16 g)

Side Effects/Toxicities
· Acute adrenal insufficiency
· Anorexia
· Diarrhea
· Dizziness
· Hemorrhagic cystitis
· Hypertension
· Lethargy
· Nausea and vomiting
· Sedation
· Vertigo
· Visual disturbances

Special Considerations
· Discontinue the drug in cases of sepsis, shock, or severe trauma
· Corticosteroids and mineralocorticoids may have to be administered

Mitoxantrone HCl · Dihydroxy-Anthracenedione Dihydrochloride, Novantrone

Drug Classification

Antitumor antibiotic

Mechanism

- Intercalates with DNA
- Inhibits the action of the enzyme DNA topoisomerase II
- Produces protein-associated double-strand breaks
- Cell cycle–nonspecific

Administration

- IV push, IV infusion

Therapeutic Use

- ALL
- Breast
- Ovarian

Usual Dose and Schedule

- Combination regimen: 10–14 mg/m^2 every 3 weeks
- Induction: 12 mg/m^2 on days 1 to 3
- Consolidation: 12 mg/m^2 on days 1 and 2, beginning approximately 6 weeks after final induction

Side Effects/Toxicities

- Alopecia
- Anemia
- Cardiac toxicity
- Leukopenia
- Nausea and vomiting
- Stomatitis
- Thrombocytopenia

Special Considerations

- Cardiac toxicity is probably less than with doxorubicin, but prior anthracycline, chest irradiation, or underlying cardiac disease increases risk

Nandrolone · Durabolin

Drug Classification
Hormonal agent, androgen

Mechanism
· Exact mechanism of action is unknown

Administration
· IM

Therapeutic Use
· Breast
· Protein anabolism
· Refractory anemia

Usual Dose and Schedule

· 100 mg IM 3 times weekly; 25–50 mg IM 3 times weekly; 50–100 mg IM weekly

Side Effects/Toxicities
· Alopecia
· Amenorrhea
· Anxiety
· Change in libido
· Clitoral hypertrophy
· Deepening of the voice
· Depression
· Headache
· Masculinism
· Sodium retention

Special Considerations
· None

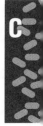

Octreotide · Sandostatin

Drug Classification
Hypothalamic peptide

Mechanism
• Mimics the action of somatostatin that naturally inhibits the release of a variety of endocrine polypeptide hormones, including growth hormone, secretin, motilin, pancreatic polypeptide, glucagon, gastric inhibitory peptide, and insulin

Administration
• SC in areas of body fat

Therapeutic Use
• Malignant carcinoid syndrome
• Suppresses secretory symptoms of neuroendocrine tumors of the gut
• Vasoactive intestinal peptide tumors

Usual Dose and Schedule

• 50 μg once or twice daily, titrated to 100–600 μg/day in 2 or 3 fractions

Side Effects/Toxicities
• Abdominal pain
• "Bloated" stomach sensation
• Constipation
• Diarrhea
• Erythema at injection site
• Flatulence
• Nausea
• Rectal spasms

Special Considerations
• None

Paclitaxel · Taxol

Drug Classification
Mitotic inhibitor

Mechanism
- Induces stable bundles of microtubules
- Prevents transition from G_0 phase to S phase

Administration
- IV infusion

Therapeutic Use
- Breast
- Malignant melanoma
- Ovarian

Usual Dose and Schedule

- Routine use: 135–250 mg/m^2 as a 24-hour continuous infusion administered every 3 weeks
- High dose: 250 mg/m^2 every 3 weeks

Side Effects/Toxicities
- Alopecia
- Bradycardia
- Diarrhea
- Dysgeusia
- Flulike symptoms
- Granulocytopenia
- Hypersensitivity reactions
- Mucositis
- Nausea and vomiting
- Peripheral neuropathy
- Phlebitis
- Rash

Special Considerations
- Anaphylactic reactions can be minimized with pretreatment with antihistamines and corticosteroids and by prolonging the infusion rate to 24 hours
- Drug must be administered with a 0.2-μm in-line filter

Pentostatin · 2′-Deoxycoformycin, Nipent

Drug Classification
Antimetabolite

Mechanism
· Irreversible inhibitor of the enzyme adenosine deaminase
· Adenosine deaminase inhibition results in inhibition of DNA synthesis

Administration
· Short IV infusion, continuous IV infusion

Therapeutic Use
· ALL
· Adult T-cell leukemia
· CLL
· Hairy cell leukemia
· Mycosis fungoides

Usual Dose and Schedule

· 4–5 mg/m^2/week for 3 consecutive weeks

Side Effects/Toxicities
· Dry skin
· Fatigue
· Granulocytopenia
· Hepatotoxicity
· Keratoconjunctivitis
· Lethargy
· Nausea and vomiting
· Nephrotoxicity

Special Considerations
· Adequate renal function must be ensured before drug administration
· Patients with severe preexisting infections should not receive the drug

Plicamycin · Aureolic Acid, Mithracin, Mithramycin

Drug Classification
Antitumor antibiotic

Mechanism
• Interrupts DNA-directed RNA synthesis
• Produces hypocalcemia

Administration
• IV infusion (4–7 hours)

Therapeutic Use
• Disseminated embryonal cell carcinoma of the testis
• Germ cell tumor
• Hypercalcemia of malignancy

Usual Dose and Schedule

• Testicular tumor: 25–35 μg/kg for 8–10 days; may repeat at monthly intervals
• Hypercalcemia: 25 μg/kg × 3–4 days

Side Effects/Toxicities
• Anorexia
• Diarrhea
• Epistaxis
• Facial flushing
• Hemorrhage
• Hepatotoxicity
• Hypocalcemia
• Metallic taste
• Nausea and vomiting
• Nephrotoxicity
• Thrombocytopenia

Special Considerations
• Administration can cause severe coagulopathy

Prednisone · Apo-Prednisone, Deltasone

Drug Classification
Corticosteroid

Mechanism
· Diverse physiologic effects
· Steroid-induced inhibition of glucose transport or phosphorylation

Administration
· PO

Therapeutic Use
· Leukemia
· Lymphoma

Usual Dose and Schedule

· 40–100 mg/m^2/day

Side Effects/Toxicities
· Cataracts
· Cushingoid syndrome
· GI bleeding
· Hyperglycemia
· Immunosuppression
· Increased ocular pressure

Special Considerations
· None

Prednisolone · Cortalone, Delta-Cortef

Drug Classification
Corticosteroid

Mechanism
- Diverse physiologic effects
- Steroid-induced inhibition of glucose transport or phosphorylation

Administration
- PO

Therapeutic Use
- Leukemia
- Lymphoma

Usual Dose and Schedule
- 40–60 mg/m^2/day

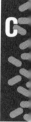

Side Effects/Toxicities
- Cataracts
- Cushingoid syndrome
- GI bleeding
- Hyperglycemia
- Immunosuppression
- Increased ocular pressure

Special Considerations
- None

Prednisolone Sodium · Hydeltrasol, Solu-Prednisolone

Drug Classification
Corticosteroid

Mechanism
- Diverse physiologic effects
- Steroid-induced inhibition of glucose transport or phosphorylation

Administration
- IM, IV

Therapeutic Use
- Acute leukemias
- Chronic leukemias

Usual Dose and Schedule

- 40–60 mg/m^2/day

Side Effects/Toxicities
- Cataracts
- Cushingoid syndrome
- GI bleeding
- Hyperglycemia
- Immunosuppression
- Increased ocular pressure

Special Considerations
- None

Procarbazine · Matulane

Drug Classification
Miscellaneous agent

Mechanism
- Forms several metabolites that have cytotoxic activity
- Produces chromosomal breakage
- Inhibits DNA, RNA, and protein synthesis

Administration
- PO, IV

Therapeutic Use
- Brain tumor
- Bronchogenic carcinoma
- Hodgkin's disease
- Malignant melanoma
- Multiple myeloma
- NHL

Usual Dose and Schedule

- MOPP combination: 100 mg/m^2/day PO for 14 days
- Single agent: 50–200 mg/day for 10–20 days
- Intermittent infusion: 300–1000 mg/m^2

Side Effects/Toxicities
- Alopecia
- Amenorrhea
- Anemia
- Anorexia
- Ataxia
- Azoospermia
- Diarrhea
- Diplopia
- Dizziness
- Flulike syndrome
- Headache
- Nausea and vomiting
- Neuropathies
- Nystagmus
- Papilledema
- Paresthesias
- Photophobia
- Pruritus
- Retinal hemorrhage
- Thrombocytopenia

Special Considerations
- Many food and drug interactions are possible. Patients should avoid ethanol, tyramine-rich foods (wine, cheese, bananas), sympathomimetic agents, tricyclic antidepressants, and CNS depressants.

Sargramostim · Granulocyte-Macrophage Colony–Stimulating Factor (GM-CSF), Leukine, Leukomax, Prokine

Drug Classification
Immunoregulating agent

Mechanism
- Stimulates granulocyte and monocyte proliferation

Administration
- IV

Therapeutic Use
- Acceleration of myeloid recovery in patients with NHL, ALL, Hodgkin's disease undergoing autologous BMT

Usual Dose and Schedule

- 250 μg/m^2/day for 21 days as a 2–4 hour infusion beginning 2–4 hours after autologous BMT

Side Effects/Toxicities
- Bone pain
- Capillary leak syndrome
- Fever
- Fluid retention
- Headache
- Hypotension
- Hypoxia
- Pericarditis
- Redness at injection site
- Venous thrombosis

Special Considerations
- None

Streptozocin · Streptozotocin, Zanosar

Drug Classification
Nitrosoureas

Mechanism
- Cross-links DNA to DNA
- Inhibits DNA synthesis
- Cell cycle–nonspecific

Administration
- IV push, IV infusion, intraperitoneal, intraarterial

Therapeutic Use
- Beta pancreatic islet cell tumors
- Gallbladder
- Hodgkin's disease
- Non–beta pancreatic islet cell tumors
- Non–small cell lung
- Oral cavity
- Synovial sarcoma
- Zollinger-Ellison tumors

Usual Dose and Schedule
- Single agent: 1.0–1.5 $g/m^2 \times 6$ consecutive weekly doses
- Combination regimen: 500 mg/m^2 or 1.0 g/m^2 for 5 consecutive days

Side Effects/Toxicities
- Altered glucose metabolism
- Burning sensation at injection site
- Duodenal ulcers
- Hepatotoxicity
- Nausea and vomiting
- Nephrotoxicity

Special Considerations
- 30–60 minute infusion recommended to reduce local pain and burning sensation around the vein
- Avoid extravasation
- Have 50% glucose available to treat sudden hypoglycemia

C

Tamoxifen · Nolvadex

Drug Classification
Nonsteroidal antiestrogen

Mechanism
- Estrogen antagonist that blocks estrogen receptors in most, but not all, hormonal tissues
- Produces cytostatic effects in hormonally responsive tumor tissues

Administration
- PO

Therapeutic Use
- Breast
- Endometrial
- Melanoma
- Prostate, Stage D
- Renal cell

Usual Dose and Schedule
- 10–20 mg b.i.d.

Side Effects/Toxicities
- Bone pain
- Cataracts
- Depression
- Dizziness
- Headache
- Hot flashes
- Leg cramps
- Lethargy
- Menstrual irregularities
- Nausea
- Peripheral edema
- Retinal hemorrhage
- Skin rash
- Vaginal bleeding

Special Considerations
- Hypercalcemia may be seen during initial therapy

Teniposide · Vumon

Drug Classification
Mitotic inhibitor

Mechanism
- Inhibits topoisomerase II
- Produces DNA double-strand breaks
- Cell cycle–specific

Administration
- IV infusion

Therapeutic Use
- ALL
- Neuroblastoma
- NHL

Usual Dose and Schedule

- 45–60 mg/m^2/day $\times$ 5 every 21 days
- 120–160 mg/m^2 on days 1, 3, and 5 every 21 days
- 100 mg/m^2 on days 1 and 2 every 3 weeks
- 100 mg/m^2/week

Side Effects/Toxicities
- Chemical phlebitis
- Hemolytic anemia
- Hypersensitivity reaction
- Hypertension
- Hypotension
- Leukopenia
- Thrombocytopenia

Special Considerations
- Possible vesicant
- Hypersensitivity reactions can occur and are often prevented with pretreatment administration of diphenhydramine and hydrocortisone
- Hypotension can be reduced by prolonging the infusion time

Testolactone · Teslac

Drug Classification
Hormonal agent, androgen

Mechanism
· Exact mechanism of action unknown

Administration
· PO

Therapeutic Use
· Androgen-responsive breast cancer in postmenopausal females

Usual Dose and Schedule
· 250 mg q.i.d.

Side Effects/Toxicities
· Alopecia
· Amenorrhea
· Anxiety
· Change in libido
· Clitoral hypertrophy
· Deepening of the voice
· Depression
· Headache
· Masculinization
· Sodium retention

Special Considerations
· None

Testosterone Cypionate · Andronate, DEPO-Testosterone

Drug Classification
Hormonal agent, androgen

Mechanism
· Exact mechanism of action unknown

Administration
· IM

Therapeutic Use
· Androgen-responsive breast cancer in postmenopausal females

Usual Dose and Schedule

· 200–400 mg every 2–4 weeks

Side Effects/Toxicities
· Alopecia
· Amenorrhea
· Anxiety
· Change in libido
· Clitoral hypertrophy
· Deepening of the voice
· Depression
· Headache
· Masculinism
· Sodium retention

Special Considerations
· Inject deep IM to minimize pain at injection site

Testosterone Enanthate · Everone, Malogex, Testrin PA

Drug Classification
Hormonal agent, androgen

Mechanism
· Exact mechanism of action unknown

Administration
· IM

Therapeutic Use
· Androgen-responsive breast cancer in postmenopausal females

Usual Dose and Schedule

· 200–400 mg every 2–4 weeks

Side Effects/Toxicities
· Alopecia
· Amenorrhea
· Anxiety
· Change in libido
· Clitoral hypertrophy
· Deepening of the voice
· Depression
· Headache
· Masculinism
· Sodium retention

Special Considerations
· Inject deep IM to minimize pain at injection site

Testosterone Propionate · Malogen, Testex

Drug Classification
Hormonal agent, androgen

Mechanism
· Exact mechanism of action unknown

Administration
· IM

Therapeutic Use
· Androgen-responsive breast cancer in postmenopausal females

Usual Dose and Schedule

· 50–100 mg 3 times a week

Side Effects/Toxicities
· Alopecia
· Amenorrhea
· Anxiety
· Change in libido
· Clitoral hypertrophy
· Deepening of the voice
· Depression
· Headache
· Masculinism
· Sodium retention

Special Considerations
· Inject deep IM to minimize pain at injection site

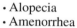

Thioguanine · Tabloid

Drug Classification

Antimetabolite

Mechanism

· Inhibits nucleotide synthesis
· S phase–specific

Administration

· PO, IV, intraperitoneal

Therapeutic Use

· ALL
· AML
· CML

Usual Dose and Schedule

· 2 to 2.5 mg/kg/day

Side Effects/Toxicities

· Anemia
· Anorexia
· Diarrhea
· Hepatotoxicity
· Hyperuricemia
· Leukopenia
· Nausea and vomiting
· Stomatitis
· Thrombocytopenia
· Unsteady gait

Special Considerations

· None

Thiotepa · TESPA, Triethylenethiophosphoramide

Drug Classification
Alkylating agent

Mechanism
- Produces chain breaks in DNA
- Cell cycle–nonspecific

Administration
- IV, intratumor, intravesicular, intracavitary

Therapeutic Use
- Bladder
- Breast
- Hodgkin's disease
- Leukemia
- Lymphoma
- Lymphosarcoma
- Ovarian

Usual Dose and Schedule

- IV initial dose: 0.4 mg/kg; maintenance dose: 0.3 mg/kg every 1–4 weeks
- Intratumor initial dose: 0.6–0.8 mg/kg; maintenance dose 0.07–0.8 mg/kg every 1–4 weeks
- Intravesical: 30–60 mg or 10–30 mg/m^2 in 30–60 ml distilled water once a week for 3–4 weeks or 6–8 weeks
- Intracavitary: 0.6–0.8 mg/kg

Side Effects/Toxicities
- Allergic reaction
- Dizziness
- Headache
- Leukopenia
- Nausea and vomiting
- Paresthesias
- Thrombocytopenia

Special Considerations
- Dose should be reduced for patients with renal disease

Vinblastine · Velban, Velbe

Drug Classification
Mitotic inhibitor

Mechanism
- Binds to tubulin
- Inhibits mitotic spindle formation
- M phase–specific

Administration
- IV push, continuous IV infusion

Therapeutic Use
- Bladder
- Breast
- Choriocarcinoma
- CML
- Histiocytosis X
- Hodgkin's disease
- NHL
- Renal cell carcinoma
- Testicular

Usual Dose and Schedule

- Dose range is 0.1–0.5 mg/kg/week. Start patients on a low dose of 8 mg/m^2 and work up in 0.05-mg/kg increments (maximal single dose 18.5 mg/m^2)

Side Effects/Toxicities
- Abdominal pain
- Adynamic ileus
- Alopecia
- Constipation
- Corneal irritation
- Depression
- Headache
- Jaw pain
- Leukopenia
- Malaise
- Muscle pain
- Nausea and vomiting
- Orthostatic hypotension
- Paresthesias
- Peripheral neuropathy
- Photosensitivity
- Rash
- Raynaud's phenomenon
- Seizures
- Stomatitis
- Tachycardia
- Urine retention

Special Considerations
- Avoid extravasation

Vincristine · Oncovin

Drug Classification
Mitotic inhibitor

Mechanism
- Arrests cell division in metaphase
- Decreases protein and RNA synthesis
- Cell cycle–specific

Administration
- IV push, IV infusion

Therapeutic Use
- ALL
- Breast
- Ewing's sarcoma
- Hodgkin's disease
- Neuroblastoma
- NHL
- Rhabdomyosarcoma
- Wilms' tumor

Usual Dose and Schedule
- 1–2 mg/m^2 (maximum 2.0–2.4 mg) IV weekly

Side Effects/Toxicities
- Anorexia
- Constipation
- Fatigue
- Fever
- Extravasation
- Jaw pain
- Paralytic ileus
- SIADH

Special Considerations
- Avoid extravasation
- Stool softeners or high-fiber diet may prevent severe constipation
- Neurotoxicity is cumulative; perform neurologic evaluation with each dose; underlying neurologic disease accentuates vincristine's effect

Vindesine · Desacetyl Vinblastine Amide, Eldisine

Drug Classification

Mitotic inhibitor

Mechanism

· Disrupts the mitotic spindle
· Cell cycle–specific

Administration

· Slow IV push, continuous IV infusion

Therapeutic Use

· ALL
· Breast
· CML (blast crisis)
· Colorectal
· Esophageal
· Hodgkin's disease
· Lung
· Malignant glioma
· Melanoma
· NHL

Usual Dose and Schedule

· 2–3 mg/m^2 IV bolus (2–3 min) for induction, then every 2 weeks

Side Effects/Toxicities

· Abdominal cramping
· Alopecia
· Cellulitis
· Cortical blindness
· Distal paresthesias
· Interstitial pneumonitis
· Loss of DTRs
· Maculopapular rash
· Nausea and vomiting
· Neutropenia
· Paralytic ileus
· Phlebitis
· Proximal muscle weakness
· Stomatitis
· Thrombocytopenia

Special Considerations

· Avoid extravasation
· Do not give concomitantly with vincristine or vinblastine

Vinorelbine Tartrate · Navelbine

Drug Classification
Vinca alkaloid

Mechanism
· Interferes with microtubule assembly
· Inhibits mitosis at metaphase

Administration
· IV (6–10 minute IV infusion)

Therapeutic Use
· Non–small cell lung

Usual Dose and Schedule

· 30 mg/m^2 weekly

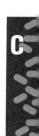

Side Effects/Toxicities
· Alopecia
· Constipation
· Diarrhea
· Dyspnea
· Extravasation
· Fatigue
· Granulocytopenia
· Injection site reactions
· Nausea and vomiting
· Peripheral neuropathy

Special Considerations
· Adjust dose in patients with granulocytopenia or hepatic insufficiency
· Administer into the sideport of a freely flowing IV

Bibliography

Aldesleukin

Whittington, R., & Faulds, D. (1993). Interleukin-2. A review of its pharmacological properties and therapeutic use in patients with cancer. *Drugs, 46*(3), 446–514.

Altretamine

Moore, D. H., Valea, F., Crumpler, L. S., & Fowler, W. C., Jr. (1993). Hexamethylmelamine/ altretamine as second-line therapy for epithelial ovarian carcinoma. *Gynecologic Oncology, 51*(1), 109–112.

Aminoglutethimide

Lundgren, S. (1992). Progestins in breast cancer treatment. A review. *Acta Oncologica, 31*(7), 709–722.

Asparaginase

Krc, I., & Krcova, V. (1991). L-Asparaginase—a reassessment. *Acta Universitatis Palackianae Olomucensis Facultatis Medicae (Praha), 129,* 57–61.

Bacillus Calmette-Guérin

Friberg, S. (1993). BCG in the treatment of superficial cancer of the bladder: A review. *Medical Oncology and Tumor Pharmacotherapy, 10*(1–2), 31–36.
Rogerson, J. W. (1994). Intravesical bacille Calmette-Guerin in the treatment of superficial transitional cell carcinoma of the bladder. *British Journal of Urology, 73*(6), 655–658.
Steg, A., Adjiman, S., & Debre, B. (1992). BCG therapy in superficial bladder tumours— complications and precautions. *European Urology, 1992, 21*(Suppl. 2), 35–40.

Bleomycin

Chisholm, R. A., Dixon, A. K., Williams, M. V., & Oliver, R. T. (1992). Bleomycin lung: The effect of different chemotherapeutic regimens. *Cancer Chemotherapy and Pharmacology, 30*(2), 158–160.
Moffett, M. J., & Ruckdeschel, J. C. (1992). Bleomycin and tetracycline in malignant pleural effusions: A review. *Seminars in Oncology, 19*(2, Suppl. 5), 59–62.
Petering, D. H., Byrnes, R. W., & Antholine, W. E. (1990). The role of redox-active metals in the mechanism of action of bleomycin. *Chemico-Biological Interactions, 1990, 73*(2–3), 133–182.

Busulfan

Buggia, I., Locatelli, F., Regazzi, M. B., & Zecca, M. (1994). Busulfan. *Annals of Pharmacotherapy, 28*(9), 1055–1062.
Vassal, G. (1994). Pharmacologically-guided dose adjustment of busulfan in high-dose chemotherapy regimens: Rationale and pitfalls. *Anticancer Research, 14*(6A), 2363–2370.

Carboplatin

Bin, P., Boddy, A. V., English, M. W., Pearson, A. D., Price, L., Tilby, M. J., & Newell, D. R. (1994). The comparative pharmacokinetics and pharmacodynamics of cisplatin and carboplatin in paediatric patients: A review. *Anticancer Research, 14*(6A), 2279–2283.
Comis, R. L. (1993). Carboplatin in the treatment of non–small cell lung cancer: A review. *Oncology, 50*(Suppl. 2), 37–41.
Cornelison, T. L., & Reed, E. (1993). Nephrotoxicity and hydration management for cisplatin, carboplatin, and ormaplatin. *Gynecologic Oncology, 50*(2), 147–158.
Hodes, T. J., Underberg, W. J., Los, G., & Beijnen, J. H. (1992). Platinum antitumour agents: A review of (bio)analysis. *Pharmaceutisch Weekblad. Scientific Edition (Utrecht), 14*(3), 61–77.
Kintzel, P. E., & Dorr, R. T. (1995). Anticancer drug renal toxicity and elimination: Dosing guidelines for altered renal function. *Cancer Treatment Reviews, 21*(1), 33–64.
Ruckdeschel, J. C. (1994). The future role of carboplatin. *Seminars in Oncology, 1994,*(5, Suppl. 12), 114–118.
Thigpen, T., Vance, R., Puneky, L., & Khansur, T. (1994). Chemotherapy in advanced ovarian carcinoma: Current standards of care based on randomized trials. *Gynecologic Oncology, 55*(3, Pt. 2), S97–S107.
Weidmann, B., Mulleneisen, N., Bojko, P., & Niederle, N. (1994). Hypersensitivity reactions to carboplatin. Report of two cases, review of the literature, and discussion of diagnostic procedures and management. *Cancer, 73*(8), 2218–2222.
Weiss, R. B., & Christian, M. C. (1993). New cisplatin analogues in development. A review. *Drugs, 46*(3), 360–377.

Carmustine

Paoletti, P., Butti, G., Knerich, R., Gaetani, P., & Assietti, R. (1990). Chemotherapy for malignant gliomas of the brain: A review of ten-years experience. *Acta Neurochirurgica, 103*(1–2), 35–46.

Chlorambucil

Counihan, T. J., & Feighery, C. (1991). Immunosuppressive therapy in autoimmune disease—a review. *Irish Journal of Medical Science, 160*(7), 199–205.
Giles, F. J., Smith, M. P., & Goldstone, A. H. (1990). Chlorambucil lung toxicity. *Acta Haematologica, 83*(3), 156–158.
Jaiyesimi, I. A., Kantarjian, H. M., & Estey, E. H. (1993). Advances in therapy for hairy cell leukemia. A review. *Cancer, 72*(1), 5–16.

Chlorotrianisene

Moore, S. R., Reinberg, Y., & Zhang, G. (1992). Small cell carcinoma of prostate: Effectiveness of hormonal versus chemotherapy. *Urology, 39*(5), 411–416.

Cisplatin

Cooley, M. E., Davis, L., & Abrahm, J. (1994). Cisplatin: A clinical review. Part II—Nursing assessment and management of side effects of cisplatin. *Cancer Nursing, 17*(4), 283–293.
Cooley, M. E., Davis, L. E., DeStefano, M., & Abrahm, J. (1994). Cisplatin: A clinical review. Part I—Current uses of cisplatin and administration guidelines. *Cancer Nursing, 1994, 17*(3), 173–184.
Fram, R. J. (1992). Cisplatin and platinum analogues: Recent advances. *Current Opinion in Oncology, 4*(6), 1073–1079.
Lichtman, S. M., Buchholtz, M., Marino, J., Schulman, P., Allen, S. L., Weiselberg, L., Budman, D., DeMarco, L., Schuster, M., & Lovecchio, J. (1992). Use of cisplatin for elderly patients. *Age and Ageing, 21*(3), 202–204.
Pinzani, V., Bressolle, F., Haug, I. J., Galtier, M., Blayac, J. P., & Balmes, P. (1994). Cisplatin-induced renal toxicity and toxicity-modulating strategies: A review. *Cancer Chemotherapy and Pharmacology, 35*(1), 1–9.

Cladribine

Bryson, H. M., & Sorkin, E. M. (1993). Cladribine. A review of its pharmacodynamic and pharmacokinetic properties and therapeutic potential in haematological malignancies. *Drugs, 46*(5), 872–894.
Guchelaar, H. J., Richel, D. J., & Schaafsma, M. R. (1994). Clinical and toxicological aspects of the antineoplastic drug cladribine: A review. *Annals of Hematology, 69*(5), 223–230.
Saven, A., & Piro, L. D. (1994). 2-Chlorodeoxy-adenosine: A newer purine analog active in the treatment of indolent lymphoid malignancies. *Annals of Internal Medicine, 120*(9), 784–791.

Cyclophosphamide

Copelan, E. A. (1992). Conditioning regimens for allogeneic bone marrow transplantation. *Blood Reviews, 6*(4), 234–242.

deVries, C. R., & Freiha, F. S. (1990). Hemorrhagic cystitis: A review. *Journal of Urology, 143*(1), 1–9.

Levine, L. A., & Jarrard, D. F. (1993). Treatment of cyclophosphamide-induced hemorrhagic cystitis with intravesical carboprost tromethamine. *Journal of Urology, 149*(4), 719–723.

McCune, W. J., Vallance, D. K., & Lynch, J. P., 3rd. (1994). Immunosuppressive drug therapy. *Current Opinion in Rheumatology, 6*(3), 262–272.

Miller, L. J., Chandler, S. W., & Ippoliti, C. M. (1994). Treatment of cyclophosphamide-induced hemorrhagic cystitis with prostaglandins. *Annals of Pharmacotherapy, 28*(5), 590–594.

Santos, G. W. (1993). Busulfan and cyclophosphamide versus cyclophosphamide and total body irradiation for marrow transplantation in chronic myelogenous leukemia—a review. *Leukemia and Lymphoma, 11*(Suppl. 1), 201–204.

Cytarabine

Hiddemann, W. (1991). Cytosine arabinoside in the treatment of acute myeloid leukemia: The role and place of high-dose regimens. *Annals of Hematology, 62*(4), 119–128.

Reykdal, S., Sham, R., & Kouides, P. (1995). Cytarabine-induced pericarditis: A case report and review of the literature of the cardio-pulmonary complications of cytarabine therapy. *Leukemia Research, 19*(2), 141–144.

Richards, C., & Wujcik, D. (1992). Cutaneous toxicity associated with high-dose cytosine arabinoside. *Oncology Nursing Forum, 19*(8), 1191–1195.

Wells, R. J., Woods, W. G., Lampkin, B. C., Nesbit, M. E., Lee, J. W., Buckley, J. D., Versteeg, C., & Hammond, G. D. (1993). Impact of high-dose cytarabine and asparaginase intensification on childhood acute myeloid leukemia: A report from the Children's Cancer Group. *Journal of Clinical Oncology, 11*(3), 538–545.

Dacarbazine

Steffens, T. A., Bajorin, D. F., Chapman, P. B., Lovett, D. R., Cody-Johnson, B. V., Templeton, M. A., Heelan, R. T., Wong, G. Y., Portlock, C. S., & Oettgen, H. F. (1991). A phase II trial of high-dose cisplatin and dacarbazine. Lack of efficacy of high-dose, cisplatin-based therapy for metastatic melanoma. *Cancer, 68*(6), 1230–1237.

Dactinomycin

Cohen, I. J., Loven, D., Schoenfeld, T., Sandbank, J., Kaplinsky, C., Yaniv, Y., Jaber, L., & Zaizov, R. (1991). Dactinomycin potentiation of radiation pneumonitis: A forgotten interaction. *Pediatric Hematology and Oncology, 8*(2), 187–192.

Daunorubicin

Boulad, F., & Kernan, N. A. (1993). Treatment of childhood acute nonlymphoblastic leukemia: A review. *Cancer Investigation, 11*(5), 534–553.

Dexamethasone

Routh, A., Khansur, T., Hickman, B. T., & Bass, D. (1994). Management of brain metastases: Past, present, and future. *Southern Medical Journal, 87*(12), 1218–1226.

Wolkowitz, O. M. (1994). Prospective controlled studies of the behavioral and biological effects of exogenous corticosteroids. *Psychoneuroendocrinology, 19*(3), 233–255.

Diethylstilbesterol

Giusti, R. M., Iwamoto, K., & Hatch, E. E. (1995). Diethylstilbestrol revisited: A review of the long-term health effects. *Annals of Internal Medicine, 122*(10), 778–788.

Macarthur, C., Foran, P. J., & Bailar, J. C., 3rd. (1995). Qualitative assessment of studies included in a meta-analysis: DES and the risk of pregnancy loss. *Journal of Clinical Epidemiology, 48*(6), 739–747.

Venner, P. M. (1990). Therapeutic options in treatment of advanced carcinoma of the prostate. *Seminars in Oncology, 17*(6, Suppl. 9), 73–77.

Doxorubicin

Allen, T. M. (1994). Long-circulating (sterically stabilized) liposomes for targeted drug delivery. *Trends in Pharmacological Sciences, 15*(7), 215–220.

Barrett, R. J., Blessing, J. A., Homesley, H. D., Twiggs, L., & Webster, K. D. (1993). Circadian-timed combination doxorubicin-cisplatin chemotherapy for advanced endometrial carcinoma. A phase II study of the Gynecologic Oncology Group. *American Journal of Clinical Oncology, 16*(6), 494–496.

Keizer, H. G., Pinedo, H. M., Schuurhuis, G. J., & Joenje, H. (1990). Doxorubicin (Adriamycin): A critical review of free radical–dependent mechanisms of cytotoxicity. *Pharmacology and Therapeutics, 47*(2), 219–231.

Lown, J. W. (1993). Anthracycline and anthraquinone anticancer agents: Current status and recent developments. *Pharmacology and Therapeutics, 60*(2), 185–214.

Namer, M. (1993). Anthracyclines in the adjuvant treatment of breast cancer. *Drugs, 45*(Suppl. 2), 4–9.

Tritton, T. R. (1991). Cell surface actions of Adriamycin. *Pharmacology and Therapeutics, 49*(3), 293–309.

Epirubicin

Mouridsen, H. T., Alfthan, C., Bastholt, L., Bergh, J., Dalmark, M., Eksborg, S., Hellsten, S., Kjaer, M., Peterson, C., & Skovsgard, T. (1990). Current status of epirubicin (Farmorubicin) in the treatment of solid tumours. *Acta Oncologica, 29*(3), 257–285.

Plosker, G. L., & Faulds, D. (1993). Epirubicin. A review of its pharmacodynamic and pharmaco-kinetic properties, and therapeutic use in cancer chemotherapy. *Drugs, 45*(5), 788–856.

Epoetin Alfa

Krantz, S. B. (1990). Review of patients' responses to epoetin alfa therapy. *Pharmacotherapy, 10*(2, Pt. 2), 15S–21S.

Markham, A., & Bryson, H. M. (1995). Epoetin alfa. A review of its pharmacodynamic and pharmacokinetic properties and therapeutic use in nonrenal applications. *Drugs, 49*(2), 232–254.

Rieger, P. T., & Haeuber, D. (1995). A new approach to managing chemotherapy-related anemia: Nursing implications of epoetin alfa. *Oncology Nursing Forum, 22*(1), 71–81.

Estradiol

Balfour, J. A., & McTavish, D. (1992). Transdermal estradiol. A review of its pharmacological profile, and therapeutic potential in the prevention of postmenopausal osteoporosis. *Drugs and Aging, 2*(6), 487–507.

Estrogen

Grady, D., Gebretsadik, T., Kerlikowske, K., Ernster, V., & Petitti, D. (1995). Hormone replacement therapy and endometrial cancer risk: A meta-analysis. *Obstetrics and Gynecology, 85*(2), 304–313.

Lupulescu, A. (1995). Estrogen use and cancer incidence: A review. *Cancer Investigation, 13*(3), 287–295.

McKeon, V. A. (1994). Hormone replacement therapy: Evaluating the risks and benefits. *Journal of Obstetric, Gynecologic, and Neonatal Nursing, 23*(8), 647–657.

Muss, H. B. (1992). Endocrine therapy for advanced breast cancer: A review. *Breast Cancer Research and Treatment, 21*(1), 15–26.

Etoposide

Bishop, J. F. (1991). Etoposide in the management of leukemia: A review. *Seminars in Oncology, 18*(1, Suppl. 2), 62–69.

Bonomi, P. (1991). Recent advances in etoposide therapy for non–small cell lung cancer. *Cancer, 67*(1, Suppl.), 254–259.

de Souza, P., Friedlander, M., Wilde, C., Kirsten, F., & Ryan, M. (1994). Hypersensitivity reactions to etoposide. A report of three cases and review of the literature. *American Journal of Clinical Oncology, 17*(5), 387–389.

Henwood, J. M., & Brogden, R. N. (1990). Etoposide. A review of its pharmacodynamic and pharmacokinetic properties, and therapeutic potential in combination chemotherapy of cancer. *Drugs, 39*(3), 438–490.

Filgrastim

Frampton, J. E., Lee, C. R., & Faulds, D. (1994). Filgrastim. A review of its pharmacological properties and therapeutic efficacy in neutropenia. *Drugs, 48*(5), 731–760.

Floxuridine

Leichman, C. G. (1994). Prolonged infusion of fluorinated pyrimidines in gastrointestinal malignancies: A review of recent clinical trials. *Cancer Investigation, 12*(2), 166–175.

Fludarabine Phosphate

Ross, S. R., McTavish, D., & Faulds, D. (1993). Fludarabine. A review of its pharmacological properties and therapeutic potential in malignancy. *Drugs, 45*(5), 737–759.

5-Fluorouracil

Anand, A. J. (1994). Fluorouracil cardiotoxicity. *Annals of Pharmacotherapy, 28*(3), 374–378.

Chrisp, P., & McTavish, D. (1991). Levamisole/fluorouracil. A review of their pharmacology and adjuvant therapeutic use in colorectal cancer. *Drugs and Aging, 1*(4), 317–337.

Hansen, R. M. (1991). 5-Fluorouracil by protracted venous infusion: A review of recent clinical studies. *Cancer Investigation, 9*(6), 637–642.

Leichman, C. G. (1994). Prolonged infusion of fluorinated pyrimidines in gastrointestinal malignancies: A review of recent clinical trials. *Cancer Investigation, 12*(2), 166–175.

Parker, W. B., & Cheng, Y. C. (1990). Metabolism and mechanism of action of 5-fluorouracil. *Pharmacology and Therapeutics, 48*(3), 381–395.

Pazdur, R., Jackson, D., Shepherd, B., Saddler, D., Font, L., McCardell, M., Myers, P., & Schmidt, S. (1991). 5-Fluorouracil and recombinant interferon alfa-2a: Review of activity and toxicity in advanced colorectal carcinomas. *Oncology Nursing Forum, 18*(1, Suppl.), 11–17.

Peters, G. J., & van Groeningen, C. J. (1991). Clinical relevance of biochemical modulation of 5-fluorouracil. *Annals of Oncology, 2*(7), 469–480.

Wils, J. A. (1992). High-dose fluorouracil: A new perspective in the treatment of colorectal cancer? *Seminars in Oncology, 19*(2, Suppl. 3), 126–130.

Flutamide

Brogden, R. N., & Chrisp, P. (1991). Flutamide. A review of its pharmacodynamic and pharmacokinetic properties, and therapeutic use in advanced prostatic cancer. *Drugs and Aging, 1*(2), 104–115.

Oosterlinck, W., & Mast, P. (1994). Total androgen blockade in the treatment of hormone-resistant metastasized prostate carcinoma. A literature review. *Acta Urologica Belgica, 62*(1), 67–71.

Gallium Nitrate

Todd, P. A., & Fitton, A. (1991). Gallium nitrate. A review of its pharmacological properties and therapeutic potential in cancer related hypercalcaemia. *Drugs, 2*(2), 261–273.

Goserelin

Brogden, R. N., & Faulds, D. (1995). Goserelin. A review of its pharmacodynamic and pharmacokinetic properties and therapeutic efficacy in prostate cancer. *Drugs and Aging, 6*(4), 324–343.

Chrisp, P., & Goa, K. L. (1991). Goserelin. A review of its pharmacodynamic and pharmacokinetic properties, and clinical use in sex hormone–related conditions. *Drugs, 41*(2), 254–288.

Shaheen, J. A., Amin, M., & Harty, J. I. (1993). Patient compliance in treatment of prostate cancer with luteinizing hormone–releasing hormone (LHRH) agonist. *Urology, 42*(5), 533–535.

Idarubicin

Berman, E. (1993). A review of idarubicin in acute leukemia. *Oncology, 7*(10), 91–98, 104.

Hollingshead, L. M., & Faulds, D. (1991). Idarubicin. A review of its pharmacodynamic and pharmacokinetic properties, and therapeutic potential in the chemotherapy of cancer. *Drugs, 42*(4), 690–719.

Ifosfamide

Dechant, K. L., Brogden, R. N., Pilkington, T., & Faulds, D. (1991). Ifosfamide/mesna. A review of its antineoplastic activity, pharmacokinetic properties and therapeutic efficacy in cancer. *Drugs, 42*(3), 428–467.

Kaijser, G. P., Beijnen, J. H., Bult, A., & Underberg, W. J. (1994). Ifosfamide metabolism and pharmacokinetics. *Anticancer Research, 14*(2A), 517–531.

Lewis, L. D. (1991). Ifosfamide pharmacokinetics. *Investigational New Drugs, 9*(4), 305–311.

Immune Globulin

Guglielmo, B. J., Wong-Beringer, A., & Linker, CA. (1994). Immune globulin therapy in allogeneic bone marrow transplant: A critical review. *Bone Marrow Transplantation, 13*(5), 499–510.

Pirofsky, B., & Kinzey, D. M. (1992). Intravenous immune globulins. A review of their uses in selected immunodeficiency and autoimmune diseases. *Drugs, 43*(1), 6–14.

Siadak, M. F., Kopecky, K., & Sullivan, K. M. (1994). Reduction in transplant-related complications in patients given intravenous immuno globulin after allogeneic marrow transplantation: *Clinical and Experimental Immunology, 97*(Suppl. 1), 53–57.

Interferon Alfa-2a

Baron, E., & Narula, S. (1990). From cloning to a commercial realization: Human alpha interferon. *Critical Reviews in Biotechnology, 10*(3), 179–190.

de Wit, R. (1992). AIDS-associated Kaposi's sarcoma and the mechanisms of interferon alpha's activity: A riddle within a puzzle. *Journal of Internal Medicine, 231*(4), 321–325.

Interferon Alfa-2b

Cooper, M. R. (1991). A review of the clinical studies of alpha-interferon in the management of multiple myeloma. *Seminars in Oncology, 18*(5, Suppl. 7), 18 –29.

Interleukin-1

Dinarello, C. A. (1993). Modalities for reducing interleukin 1 activity in disease. *Immunology Today, 14*(6), 260–264.

Dinarello, C. A. (1994). The biological properties of interleukin-1. *European Cytokine Network, 5*(6), 517–531.

Johnson, C. S. (1992). Modulation of chemotherapy antineoplastic agents with biologic agents: Enhancement of antitumor activities by interleukin-1. *Current Opinion in Oncology, 4*(6), 1108–1115.

Shintani, F., Nakaki, T., Kanba, S., Kato, R., & Asai, M. (1995). Role of interleukin-1 in stress responses. A putative neurotransmitter. *Molecular Neurobiology, 10*(1), 47–71.

Leuprolide Acetate

Chrisp, P., & Sorkin, E. M. (1991). Leuprorelin. A review of its pharmacology and therapeutic use in prostatic disorders. *Drugs and Aging, 1*(6), 487–509.

Plosker, G. L., & Brogden, R. N. (1994). Leuprorelin. A review of its pharmacology and therapeutic use in prostatic cancer, endometriosis and other sex hormone–related disorders. *Drugs, 48*(6), 930–967.

Levamisole

de Brabander, M., De Cree, J., Vandebroek, J., Verhaegen, H., & Janssen, P. A. (1992). Levamisole in the treatment of cancer: Anything new? *Anticancer Research, 12*(1), 177–187.

Chrisp, P., & McTavish, D. (1991). Levamisole/fluorouracil. A review of their pharmacology and adjuvant therapeutic use in colorectal cancer. *Drugs and Aging, 1*(4), 317–337.

Medroxyprogesterone

Chilvers, C. (1994). Breast cancer and depot-medroxyprogesterone acetate: A review. *Contraception, 49*(3), 211–222.

Kaunitz, A. M. (1994). Long-acting injectable contraception with depot medroxyprogesterone acetate. *American Journal of Obstetrics and Gynecology, 170*, 1543–1549.

Lumbiganon, P. (1994). Depot-medroxyprogesterone acetate (DMPA) and cancer of the endometrium and ovary. *Contraception, 49*(3), 203–209.

Lundgren, S. (1992). Progestins in breast cancer treatment. A review. *Acta Oncologica, 31*(7), 709–722.

Udoff, L., Langenberg, P., & Adashi, E. Y. (1995). Combined continuous hormone replacement therapy: A critical review. *Obstetrics and Gynecology, 86*(2), 306–316.

Melphalan

Samuels, B. L., & Bitran, J. D. (1995). High-dose intravenous melphalan: A review. *Journal of Clinical Oncology, 13*(7), 1786–1799.

Mercaptopurine

Pinkel, D. (1993). Intravenous mercaptopurine: Life begins at 40. *Journal of Clinical Oncology, 11*(9), 1826–1831.

Mesna

Goren, M. P. (1992). Oral mesna: A review. *Seminars in Oncology, 19*(6, Suppl. 12), 65–71.

Lewis, C. (1994). A review of the use of chemoprotectants in cancer chemotherapy. *Drug Safety, 11*(3), 153–162.

deVries, C. R., & Freiha, F. S. (1990). Hemorrhagic cystitis: A review. *Journal of Urology, 143*(1), 1–9.

Methotrexate

Grosflam, J., & Weinblatt, M. E. (1991). Methotrexate: Mechanism of action, pharmacokinetics, clinical indications, and toxicity. *Current Opinion in Rheumatology, 3*(3), 363–368.

Methylprednisolone

Nelson, D. A. (1993). Intraspinal therapy using methylprednisolone acetate. Twenty-three years of clinical controversy. *Spine, 18*(2), 278–286.

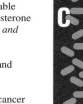

Wilkinson, H. A. (1992). Intrathecal Depo-Medrol: A literature review. *Clinical Journal of Pain, 8*(1), 49–56; discussion 57–58.

Mitomycin

Kohnoe, S., Maehara, Y., Takahashi, I., Saito, A., Okada, Y., & Sugimachi, K. (1994). Intrapericardial mitomycin C for the management of malignant pericardial effusion secondary to gastric cancer: Case report and review. *Chemotherapy, 40*(1), 57–60.

Linette, D. C., McGee, K. H., & McFarland, J. A. (1992). Mitomycin-induced pulmonary toxicity: Case report and review of the literature. *Annals of Pharmacotherapy, 26*(4), 481–484.

Mitoxantrone

Ehninger, G., Schuler, U., Proksch, B., Zeller, K. P., & Blanz, J. (1990). Pharmacokinetics and metabolism of mitoxantrone. A review. *Clinical Pharmacokinetics, 18*(5), 365–380.

Faulds, D., Balfour, J. A., Chrisp, P., & Langtry, H. D. (1991). Mitoxantrone. A review of its pharmacodynamic and pharmacokinetic properties, and therapeutic potential in the chemotherapy of cancer. *Drugs, 41*(3), 400–449.

Vogel, C. L. (1995). Combination chemotherapy with vinorelbine (Navelbine) and mitoxantrone for metastatic breast cancer: A review. *Seminars in Oncology, 22*(2, Suppl. 5), 61–65.

Octreotide

Brown, N. J. (1990). Octreotide: A long-acting somatostatin analog. *American Journal of the Medical Sciences, 300*(4), 267–273.

Gyr, K. E., & Meier, R. (1993). Pharmacodynamic effects of Sandostatin in the gastrointestinal tract. *Digestion, 54*(Suppl. 1), 14–19.

Maton, P. N. (1994). Expanding uses of octreotide. *Bailliere's Clinical Gastroenterology, 8*(2), 321–337.

Paclitaxel

Long, H. J. (1994). Paclitaxel (Taxol): A novel anticancer chemotherapeutic drug. *Mayo Clinic Proceedings, 69*(4), 341–345.

Lubejko, B. G., & Sartorius, S. E. (1993). Nursing considerations in paclitaxel (Taxol) administration. *Seminars in Oncology, 20*(4, Suppl. 3), 26–30.

Ravdin, P. M., & Valero, V. (1995). Review of docetaxel (Taxotere), a highly active new agent for the treatment of metastatic breast cancer. *Seminars in Oncology, 22*(2, Suppl. 4), 17–21.

Spencer, C. M., & Faulds, D. (1994). Paclitaxel. A review of its pharmacodynamic and pharmacokinetic properties and therapeutic potential in the treatment of cancer. *Drugs, 48*(5), 794–847.

Pentostatin

Brogden, R. N., & Sorkin, E. M. (1993). Pentostatin. A review of its pharmacodynamic and pharmacokinetic properties, and therapeutic potential in lymphoproliferative disorders. *Drugs, 46*(4), 652–677.

Kane, B. J., Kuhn, J. G., & Roush, M. K. (1992). Pentostatin: An adenosine deaminase inhibitor for the treatment of hairy cell leukemia. *Annals of Pharmacotherapy, 26*(7–8), 939–947.

Prednisolone

Sousa, F. J. (1991). The bioavailability and therapeutic effectiveness of prednisone acetate vs. prednisolone sodium phosphate: A 20-year review. *CLAO Journal, 17*(4), 282–284.

Prednisone

Kalaycioglu, M., Kavuru, M., Tuason, L., & Bolwell, B. (1995). Empiric prednisone therapy for pulmonary toxic reaction after high-dose chemotherapy containing carmustine (BCNU). *Chest, 107*(2), 482–487.

Sargramostim

Kellihan, M. J. (1993). Drug formulary review process for sargramostim and filgrastim: Focus on analysis of adverse drug reactions. *Clinical Therapeutics, 15*(5), 927–937.

Tamoxifen

Cohen, I., Altaras, M., Shapira, J., Tepper, R., & Beyth, Y. (1994). Postmenopausal tamoxifen treatment and endometrial pathology. *Obstetrical and Gynecological Survey, 49*(12), 823–829.

Gould, K., Gates, M. L., & Miaskowski, C. (1994). Breast cancer prevention: A summary of the chemoprevention trial with tamoxifen. *Oncology Nursing Forum, 21*(5), 835–840.

Jaiyesimi, I. A., Buzdar, A. U., Decker, D. A., & Hortobagyi, G. N. (1995). Use of tamoxifen for breast cancer: Twenty-eight years later. *Journal of Clinical Oncology, 13*(2), 513–529.

Wiseman, H. (1994). Tamoxifen: New membrane-mediated mechanisms of action and therapeutic advances. *Trends in Pharmacological Sciences, 15*(3), 83–89.

Teniposide

Takano, H., Kohno, K., Matsuo, K., Matsuda, T., & Kuwano, M. (1992). DNA topoisomerase–targeting antitumor agents and drug resistance. *Anti-Cancer Drugs, 3*(4), 323–330.

Hansen, H. H., Dombernowsky, P., Hansen, M., & Bork, E. (1992). Teniposide in the treatment of small cell lung cancer: A review. *Seminars in Oncology, 19*(2, Suppl. 6), 65–68.

van der Gaast, A., & Splinter, T. A. (1992). Teniposide (VM-26) in ovarian cancer: A review. *Seminars in Oncology, 19*(2, Suppl. 6), 95–97.

Testosterone

Bahrke, M. S., Yesalis, C. E., 3d, & Wright, J. E. (1990). Psychological and behavioural effects of endogenous testosterone levels and anabolic-androgenic steroids among males. A review. *Sports Medicine, 10*(5), 303–337.

Hutchinson, K. A. (1995). Androgens and sexuality. *American Journal of Medicine, 98*(1A), 111S–115S.

Vinblastine

Noble, R. L. (1990). The discovery of the vinca alkaloids—chemotherapeutic agents against cancer. *Biochemistry and Cell Biology, 68*(12), 1344–1351.

Vinorelbine

Goa, K. L., & Faulds, D. (1994). Vinorelbine. A review of its pharmacological properties and clinical use in cancer chemotherapy. *Drugs and Aging, 5*(3), 200–234.

Marty, M., Extra, J. M., Dieras, V., Giacchetti, S., Ohana, S., & Espie, M. (1992). A review of the antitumour activity of vinorelbine in breast cancer. *Drugs, 44*(Suppl. 4), 29–35; discussion 66–69.

Sorensen, J. B. (1992). Vinorelbine. A review of its antitumour activity in lung cancer. *Drugs, 44*(Suppl. 4), 60–65; discussion 66–69.

Oncologic Emergencies

Disseminated Intravascular Coagulation

Epidemiology
- Secondary condition
- Clotting suddenly occurs throughout the vascular system, followed by diffuse fibrinolysis
- Acute or chronic condition

Etiology/Risk Factors
- Acute promyelocytic leukemia
- Anaphylactic shock
- Chemotherapy
- Infection
- Massive tissue injury
- Mucin-producing tumors (e.g., ovarian, gastric)
- Prostate cancer
- Red blood cell damage

Signs and Symptoms
- Abdominal pain
- Acrocyanosis
- Ecchymosis
- Epistaxis
- Guaiac-positive stool
- Hematemesis
- Hematuria
- Hypotension
- Joint pain
- Mental confusion
- Oozing from injection sites
- Petechiae

Diagnostic Tests
- Activated PTT
- Antithrombin III
- D-dimer
- Fibrinogen level
- FSPs
- Hemoglobin
- Hematocrit
- Platelet count
- PT
- Schistocytes

Treatment
- Treat underlying cause
- Heparin therapy: 2500–5000 units q4–8h SC; 20,000–30,000 U/day by continuous infusion
- Antithrombin III concentrate: 1500–1725 units in 50 ml distilled water IV over 10 hours
- Platelet infusion
- RBC transfusion for HCT < 20
- Clotting factors: only in case of *active* bleeding
- Amicar therapy: for excessive bleeding
- Supportive therapy: hydration, oxygen

Patient Problems
- Adult respiratory distress syndrome
- Anxiety
- CNS bleeding
- Decreased circulation to hands and feet
- GI bleeding
- GU bleeding
- High risk for injury
- Hypotension
- Pulmonary microemboli
- Renal failure
- Seizures

Prognosis
- Highly variable, depending on underlying cause

Ectopic Adrenocorticotrophic Hormone (ACTH) Production

Epidemiology

- Also called *ectopic Cushing's syndrome*
- More common in males
- Age > 50 years
- Characteristic Cushing's syndrome appearance absent

Etiology/Risk Factors

- Breast
- Carcinoids
- Colon
- Ganglioma
- Islet cell tumors
- Medullary thyroid
- Melanoma
- Neuroblastoma
- Ovarian
- Pheochromocytoma
- Prostate
- Small cell lung (oat cell)
- Thymomas

Signs and Symptoms

- Anorexia
- Edema
- Elevated blood glucose
- Fatigue
- Hyperpigmentation
- Hypertension
- Hypokalemia
- Muscle wasting
- Polydipsia
- Polyuria
- Weight loss

Diagnostic Tests

- Dexamethasone suppression test
- Glucose tolerance test
- Plasma cortisol level
- Serum glucose level
- Serum potassium level
- Serum ACTH level
- 24-hour urine for free cortisol

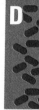
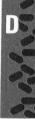

D

Treatment

- Treat the primary tumor
- Correct hypokalemia
  - Administer potassium chloride
  - IV hydration
  - Spironolactone: 100–400 mg/day
- Manage sodium and water retention
  - Administer thiazide diuretics: hydrochlorothiazide 50 mg b.i.d.; chlorthalidone 50–100 mg/day; or metolazone 2.5–5.0 mg/day
- Treat the metabolic alkalosis
- Administer adrenal enzyme inhibitors
  - Aminoglutethimide: 1 g/day divided in 4 doses. Requires supplements with hydrocortisone 40–60 mg/day (10 mg at 8 A.M., 10 mg at 5:00 P.M., and 20 mg hs) *or* dexamethasone 0.5–0.75 mg, q.i.d.
  - Mitotane: 4–8 g/day in divided doses t.i.d. or q.i.d.
  - Ketoconazole: experimental agent; dose varies from 200 mg/day to 1 g/day in divided doses
  - RU 486: experimental agent

Patient Problems

- Alterations in mobility
- CNS toxicity
- Dehydration
- Fatigue
- Hypertension
- Hypo-/hyperkalemia

Prognosis

- Variable, depending on underlying malignancy

Graft-versus-Host Disease (GVHD): Acute

Epidemiology

- Serious immune reaction
- More common with allogeneic BMT
- Seen in 80% of HLA-matched unrelated donors

Etiology/Risk Factors

- Histocompatibility differences between donor (graft) and recipient (host)
- Immunoincompetent host
- Infusion of donor marrow (graft) with immunocompetent T cells

Signs and Symptoms

- Abdominal pain
- Bullous skin lesions
- Diarrhea
- Elevated LFTs
- Fatigue
- Hepatomegaly
- Maculopapular rash
- Nausea
- Right upper quadrant pain
- Skin rash
- "Sunburned" skin
- Vomiting

Diagnostic Tests

- Liver biopsy
- Liver function tests
- Rectal biopsy
- Skin biopsy

Treatment

- Prophylaxis for allogeneic BMT: cyclosporine, methotrexate, corticosteroids, and T-cell depletion
- Established GVHD: high doses of corticosteroids, antithymocyte globulin, and monoclonal antibodies

Patient Problems

- Dehydration
- Diarrhea
- Fatigue
- Hypotension
- Impaired skin integrity
- Pain
- Perirectal abscess
- Pruritus

Prognosis

- Approximately 25% of HLA-matched siblings will die of GVHD or its complications

Graft-versus-Host Disease (GVHD): Chronic

Epidemiology
- Occurs in 50% of HLA-matched sibling BMT
- Multiorgan syndrome similar to a collagen vascular disease
- Occurs between 70 days and 15 months after BMT

Etiology/Risk Factors
- CMV infection
- Histocompatibility differences between donor (graft) and recipient (host)
- Immunoincompetent host
- Infusion of CMV-positive donor marrow
- Infusion of donor marrow (graft) with immunocompetent T cells
- Older transplant donor
- Older transplant recipient

Signs and Symptoms
- Abdominal pain
- Anxiety
- Cystitis
- Depression
- Diarrhea
- Dry eyes
- Dysphagia
- Dyspnea
- Hair loss
- Hardening of the skin
- Hyper-/hypopigmentation
- Infections
- Joint contractures
- Muscle weakness
- Neuropathy
- Painful intercourse
- Sinusitis
- Thickening of the skin
- Thrombocytopenia
- Vaginal stenosis
- Weight loss
- Wheezing
- Xerostomia

Diagnostic Tests
- Arterial blood gases
- Blood cultures
- Chest radiography
- Complete blood count
- Muscle biopsy
- Pulmonary function tests
- Schirmer's test
- Sinus radiography
- Skin biopsy
- Vaginal biopsy

Treatment
- Prednisone, cyclosporine, and/or thalidomide
- Supportive care specific to the patient's problems

Patient Problems
- Anxiety
- Body image disturbance
- Decreased mobility
- Decreased nutrition
- Depression
- Impaired gas exchange
- Impaired skin integrity
- Infection
- Pain
- Sexual dysfunction

Prognosis
- Chronic GVHD life threatening in approximately 5% of HLA-matched sibling organ recipients

Hypercalcemia

Epidemiology

- Most common oncologic emergency
- 15–20 cases per 100,000 persons
- Incidence varies with underlying cancer diagnosis

Etiology/Risk Factors

- Dehydration
- Immobilization
- Tumors metastasize to bone (breast, multiple myeloma, T-cell lymphoma, leukemia)
- Tumors secrete a PTH-related protein (squamous cell lung, squamous cell of the head and neck, hypernephroma, genitourinary)
- Tumors secrete prostaglandins
- Tumors secrete 1,25-dihydroxyvitamin D_3 (Hodgkin's disease, non-Hodgkin's lymphoma, myeloma)

Signs and Symptoms

- Anorexia
- Bradycardia
- Cardiac arrhythmias
- Coma
- Confusion
- Constipation
- Dehydration
- Fatigue
- Hyporeflexia
- Ileus
- Lethargy
- Muscle weakness
- Nausea
- Obstipation
- Obtundation
- Polydipsia
- Polyuria
- Prolonged PR interval
- Pruritus
- Psychosis
- Renal insufficiency
- Seizures
- Shortened QT interval
- Vomiting
- Weight loss
- Wide T wave

Diagnostic Tests

- BUN and creatinine
- Calculate corrected calcium: measured calcium (mg/dl) − measured albumin (g/dl) + 4.0
- ECG
- Immunoreactive PTH level
- Serum albumin
- Serum calcium level
- Serum potassium level

Treatment

- Treat the underlying cause
- Saline diuresis: 250–500 ml/hour with IV administration of furosemide 20–80 mg q2–4h
- Glucocorticoids: initial treatment with hydrocortisone 250–500 mg IV q8h followed by maintenance therapy with prednisone 10–30 mg/day
- Calcitonin: 50–100 IU followed by 4–8 IU, SC, or IM q12–24h
- Disodium etidronate: 7.5 mg/kg diluted in 250 ml normal saline, administered over at least 2 hours daily for 3–5 days
- Plicamycin: 10–50 µg/kg (usually 25 µg/kg) IV infusion; administer additional doses every 3–4 days
- Gallium nitrate: 100–200 mg/m²/day by continuous IV infusion up to 5 days
- Oral phosphate supplements: 1–3 g/day PO in divided doses
- Pamidronate: 60–90 mg IV over 24 hours
- Restrict dietary calcium
- Mobilize patient

Patient Problems

- Cardiac arrhythmias
- Confusion
- Constipation
- Dehydration
- Depression
- Fatigue
- Hypotension
- Impaired physical mobility
- Potential for injury
- Renal failure

Prognosis

- Survival depends on tumor type and specific treatment available to treat the underlying malignancy

Hyperuricemia

Epidemiology

- Acute and chronic forms
- Result of sequential catalysis of hypoxanthine and xanthine by xanthine oxidase
- Causes renal insufficiency

Etiology/Risk Factors

- High-grade lymphomas
- Leukemia
- Multiple myeloma
- Polycythemia vera
- Preexisting renal impairment
- Side effect of diuretics, antituberculosis drugs
- Squamous cell carcinoma of the head and neck

Signs and Symptoms

- Flank pain
- Gross hematuria
- Lethargy
- Nausea
- Oliguria
- Vomiting

Diagnostic Tests

- BUN and creatinine
- CT
- Renal ultrasound
- Serum electrolytes
- Serum uric acid level
- Urinalysis

Treatment

- Prevent hyperuricemia before and during chemotherapy
  - Administer allopurinol 300–900 mg/day
  - Vigorous hydration: urine output > 3L/day
  - Urine alkalinization: maintain urine pH $\geq$ 7.0 with PO or IV sodium bicarbonate, (50–100 mmol/L)
- Stop drugs that tend to elevate serum urate or that acidify urine (e.g., thiazide diuretics, salicylates)
- Consider peritoneal or hemodialysis

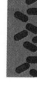

Patient Problems

- Dehydration
- Fatigue
- Fluid and electrolyte imbalances
- Impaired mobility
- Pain
- Pruritus

Prognosis

- Incidence of hyperuricemia has decreased with prophylactic treatment
- Majority of patients regain normal renal function

Intestinal Obstruction: Large Bowel

Epidemiology
- 90% of cases caused by cancer

Etiology/Risk Factors
- Primary cancer
  - Adenocarcinoma
- Metastatic disease
  - Cervix
  - Lymphoma
  - Ovary

Signs and Symptoms
- Abdominal pain
- Decreased bowel sounds
- Diarrhea/constipation (alternate)
- Marked distension
- Vomiting (late sign)

Diagnostic Tests
- Abdominal CT
- Abdominal radiography
- Serum electrolytes

Treatment

- Surgery: resection with end-to-end anastomosis or colostomy
- Radiation therapy may be used, depending on the cause of the obstruction
- Supportive therapy: nasogastric tube to relieve distension, IV hydration

Patient Problems
- Dehydration
- Infection
- Nausea
- Nutritional deficit
- Pain

Prognosis
- Variable, depending on underlying cause of obstruction

Intestinal Obstruction: Small Bowel

Epidemiology
- 90% are the result of adhesions following abdominal surgery
- Carcinoma accounts for 10–20% of obstructions

Etiology/Risk Factors
- Adhesions
- Primary cancers
  - Adenocarcinoma
  - Carcinoid
  - Lymphoma
  - Melanoma
  - Sarcoma
- Metastatic disease
  - Cervix
  - Colon/rectum
  - Gastric
  - Ovary
  - Pancreas

Signs and Symptoms
- Abdominal distension
- Abdominal pain
- Audible borborygmi
- Dehydration
- Fever
- Leukocytosis
- Obstipation
- Oliguria
- Vomiting

Diagnostic Tests
- Abdominal CT
- Abdominal radiography
- Serum amylase
- Serum electrolytes

Treatment

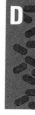

- Surgery if appropriate to relieve the obstruction
- Supportive therapy: nasogastric tube to relieve distension; long intestinal tube to provide decompression, IV hydration

Patient Problems
- Dehydration
- Infusion
- Nausea
- Nutritional deficit
- Pain

Prognosis
- Variable, depending on underlying cause of obstruction

Intracranial Hemorrhage

Epidemiology

- Two types of bleeding can occur: intracerebral hemorrhage (i.e., bleeding into the substance of the brain); subdural hematoma (bleeding into the epidural space)
- Leukocyte count > 300,000 cells/µl; patient has a 60% chance of intracranial bleed

Etiology/Risk Factors

- DIC
- Leukemia
- Sepsis
- Thrombocytopenia

Signs and Symptoms

- Intracerebral bleed
  - Change in LOC
  - Coma
  - Decerebrate posture
  - Decorticate posture
  - Hemiplegia
  - Hemisensory deficits
- Subdural hematoma
  - Brudzinski's sign
  - Change in LOC
  - Diplopia
  - Dizziness
  - Drowsiness
  - Headache
  - Hyperesthesias
  - Irritability
  - Kernig's sign
  - Nausea and vomiting
  - Nuchal rigidity
  - Opisthotonus
  - Paresis/paralysis
  - Photophobia
  - Seizures
  - Speech disorders
  - Sweating and chills
  - Vertigo

Diagnostic Tests

- CBC
- CT
- MRI
- Neurologic examination
- Platelet count
- Spinal tap (cautiously)

Treatment

- Administer platelets prophylactically during episodes of severe thrombocytopenia
- Prevent and control conditions that would increase intracranial pressure (e.g., maintain a quiet environment, bed rest, decrease stress, decrease anxiety)
- Treat seizures
- Promote cerebral vascular perfusion by maintaining blood pressure and preventing respiratory or metabolic acidosis
- Control cerebral edema with osmotic diuretics, sodium restriction, and/or dexamethasone

Patient Problems

- Anxiety
- Aphasia
- Confusion
- Contractures
- High risk for injury
- Impaired mobility
- Impaired skin integrity
- Pain
- Paralysis

Prognosis

- Recovery depends on location and extent of intracranial bleeding

Neoplastic Cardiac Tamponade

Epidemiology
- Fluid accumulates in pericardial sac
- 5–10% of patients dying with disseminated malignancy have pericardial metastasis; far fewer develop pericardial effusion
- Effusion can develop rapidly or insidiously

Etiology/Risk Factors
- Metastatic tumor invasion of the pericardium (e.g., breast, lung, lymphoma, leukemia, melanoma)
- Direct tumor invasion of or pressure on the pericardium from adjacent tumor (e.g., lung, esophageal)
- Postradiation pericarditis (e.g., Hodgkin's disease, mediastinal tumors, breast, lung)
- Cardiac tumor
- Chemotherapy-induced pericarditis
- Iatrogenic trauma (e.g., catheter perforates heart)

Signs and Symptoms
- Anxiety
- Atrial fibrillation
- Change in LOC
- Chest pain
- Chest pressure
- Cough
- Distant heart sounds
- Dyspnea
- Electrical alternans (ECG)
- Facial swelling
- Feeling of impending doom
- Hypotension
- Jugular venous distension
- Knee-chest forward-leaning position
- Hiccups
- Nausea and vomiting
- Oliguria
- Orthopnea
- Pallor
- Profuse perspiration
- Tachycardia
- Tachypnea

Diagnostic Tests
- Central venous pressure
- Chest radiography
- Echocardiogram
- ECG
- Hemodynamic monitoring
- Pulsus paradoxus

Treatment
- Volume expansion and pressor support to maintain blood pressure
- Maintain adequate oxygenation
- Pericardiocentesis under ECG and blood pressure monitoring, is done in an emergency. Preferred procedure pericardiocentesis under 2-dimensional echocardiography
- Instillation of chemotherapeutic or sclerosing agents (e.g., tetracycline, fluorouracil, thiotepa)
- Radiation therapy with radioisotopes or 2000–4000 cGy external beam may help to control effusions
- Pericardial window or pericardiectomy may be used

Patient Problems
- Altered cerebral, renal, and peripheral tissue perfusion
- Anxiety
- Decreased cardiac output
- Dyspnea
- High risk for injury
- Impaired mobility
- Pain

Prognosis
- Usual mortality 25%
- If unrecognized, mortality is 65%

Pleural Effusion

Epidemiology

- Irritation of the pleural membrane by tumor cells produces fluid in the pleural space
- Approximately 300 ml of fluid in the pleural space produces symptoms

Etiology/Risk Factors

- Breast
- GI
- Lung
- Lymphoma
- Mesothelioma
- Ovarian
- Uterine

Signs and Symptoms

- Chest pressure
- Cough
- Decreased fremitus
- Decreased or absent breath sounds
- Dullness to percussion
- Dyspnea
- Egophony
- Orthopnea
- Paroxysmal nocturnal dyspnea
- Pleuritic chest pain
- Tachypnea

Diagnostic Tests

- Chest radiography
- Thoracocentesis

Treatment

- Thoracocentesis and drainage relieves symptoms; not effective when used alone
- Cytotoxic and sclerosing agents: a wide variety of agents, including radioactive isotopes (gold, phosphorus, yttrium), talc, tetracycline, bleomycin, quinacrine, mechlorethamine, thiotepa, 5-FU, and *Corynebacterium parvum* have been used to treat pleural effusions
- Thoracotomy and pleural stripping may be tried subsequently for effusions refractory to medical management

Patient Problems

- Anxiety
- Dyspnea
- Fatigue
- Pain

Prognosis

- Approximately 95% of patients die within 1 year

Pneumocystis carinii Pneumonia

Epidemiology

- Organism is characterized as a protozoa/fungus
- Found normally in human lung
- Occurs in up to 80% of patients with AIDS without prophylaxis

Etiology/Risk Factors

- AIDS
- Cancer
- Cytotoxic drugs
- Immunosuppressive therapy
- Irradiation
- Organ transplantation
- Severe malnutrition

Signs and Symptoms

- Bibasilar crackles
- Dyspnea
- Fatigue
- Fever
- Nonproductive cough
- Tachypnea
- Weakness

Diagnostic Tests

- Chest radiography
- Gallium scan
- Needle biopsy
- Open lung biopsy
- Pulmonary function tests
- Serum LDH level
- Sputum cytology
- WBC count

Treatment

- Establish the diagnosis
- TMP-SMZ: usual dose is TMP 20 mg/kg + SMX 100 mg/kg (PO or IV for 14–21 days)
- Pentamidine isethionate: usual dose is 4 mg/kg/day (IV or IM for 14–21 days)
- Atovaquone: approved for patients with mild to moderate disease who cannot tolerate TMP-SMX or pentamidine; usual dose 750 mg t.i.d., for 21 days
- Supportive care with oxygen therapy may be indicated

Patient Problems

- Cough
- Discomfort
- Dyspnea
- Fatigue

Prognosis

- Early treatment reduces mortality rate from 100% to 25%
- Recurrences are common

Septic Shock

Epidemiology

- Occurs in 10 of every 1000 hospitalized patients
- 80% of the organisms arise from patient's endogenous flora

Etiology/Risk Factors

- Advancing age
- Corticosteroid therapy
- Granulocytopenia
- Immunodeficiency secondary to disease (i.e., leukemia, multiple myeloma, lymphoma)
- Immunodeficiency secondary to medical treatment (i.e., chemotherapy, radiation therapy, bone marrow transplantation)
- Inadequate nutrition
- Invasive procedures (catheters, lines)

Signs and Symptoms

Early
- Chills
- Discomfort
- Hyperthermia ($>$ 100.4° F) or hypothermia ($<$ 96° F)
- Malaise
- Mental status changes
- Normal BP
- Rigors
- Tachycardia
- Tachypnea
- Warm, dry skin
- Progressive
- Cool skin
- Decreasing BP
- Hyperthermia or hypothermia
- Hyperventilation
- Mental confusion
- Oliguria
- Peripheral edema
- Pulmonary congestion
- Tachycardia
- Weak, thready pulse
- Late
- Anuria
- Hyperthermia or hypothermia
- Mental confusion
- Respiratory failure
- Severe hypotension
- Tachycardia

Diagnostic Tests

- Arterial blood gases
- Blood chemistries
- Blood cultures
- Hemodynamic monitoring
- WBC count

Treatment

- Identify causative organism and treat with appropriate antibiotic therapy
- Fluid resuscitation
- Vasoactive therapy guided by hemodynamic measurements
- Scrupulous hand washing
- Protective isolation
- Reduce exposure to environmental pathogens (i.e., cook all food, no live plants in living environment)
- Monitor essential organ function (e.g., kidney, liver, lungs, heart, CNS)
- Surgical drainage of infected sites

Patient Problems

- Anxiety
- Confusion
- Decreased cardiac output
- High risk for injury
- Hypovolemia
- Impaired skin integrity
- Infection
- Renal failure
- Respiratory failure
- Weight loss

Prognosis

- Mortality rate for gram-negative sepsis 25–50%

Spinal Cord Compression

Epidemiology
- Develops in 1–10% of oncology patients
- Location: thoracic (70%), lumbosacral (20%), cervical (10%)
- Mechanisms: direct extension of tumor or metastasis

Etiology/Risk Factors
- Breast
- Kidney
- Lung
- Lymphoma
- Melanoma
- Myeloma
- Prostate

Signs and Symptoms
- Change in muscle tone
- Diarrhea or constipation
- Loss of muscle strength
- Motor weakness
- Numbness
- Pain
- Paresthesias
- Urinary retention or incontinence

Diagnostic Tests
- CT
- Lumbar puncture
- MRI
- Myelography
- Neurologic examination
- Spinal radiography

Treatment
- Surgery: indicated for patients with rapidly progressing or extremely severe neurologic deficits
- Radiation therapy: used following surgery or as the primary treatment for patients with minimal or slowly progressing symptoms
- High-dose steroids

Patient Problems
- Constipation
- Impaired mobility
- Impaired skin integrity
- Pain
- Sensory-perceptual deficits
- Urinary retention or incontinence

Prognosis
- Positive correlation between preoperative motor status and postoperative outcome
- Slowly progressive neurologic symptoms associated with better outcomes
- Posterior cord lesions associated with better prognosis than anterior cord lesions

Superior Vena Cava (SVC) Syndrome

Epidemiology
- Obstruction or compression of the SVC due to tumor or thrombosis
- Malignancy accounts for 80–90% of cases of SVC syndrome
- Occurs in 3–4% of patients with cancer
- Severity of symptoms depends on the rapidity, degree, and location of the obstruction

Etiology/Risk Factors
- Cancers
  - Breast
  - Bronchogenic carcinoma
  - Colon
  - Esophagus
  - Lymphomas
  - Mediastinal germinomas
  - NHL
  - Testicular
  - Thyroid
- Nonmalignant causes
  - Aortic aneurysm
  - Central venous catheter
  - Infectious agent
  - Substernal thyroid

Signs and Symptoms
- Anxiety
- Blurred vision
- Confusion
- Conjunctival edema
- Cough
- Cyanosis
- Difficulty putting on or removing rings
- Dyspnea
- Epistaxis
- Facial erythema
- Facial swelling
- Fullness in the arms
- Headache
- Hoarseness
- Irritability
- Lethargy
- Painless dysphagia
- Periorbital edema
- Plethora of the face
- Swelling of hands and fingers
- Tachypnea
- Throat tightness
- Tightness of the shirt collar

Diagnostic Tests
- Chest radiography
- CT
- Doppler ultrasound
- Mediastinoscopic biopsy
- Venography

Treatment
- Diuretics and high-dose steroids (dexamethasone 8–16 mg or prednisone 30–60 mg) may provide symptomatic relief
- Radiation therapy: administer before biopsy confirmation. Several daily high-dose fractions (4 Gy/day for 2 or 3 days) usually sufficient to provide temporary symptom relief
- Overall plan should be developed, after initial treatment, based on pathologic diagnosis and extent of disease

Patient Problems
- Altered cerebral perfusion
- Anxiety
- Dyspnea
- High risk for injury
- Impaired mobility
- Impaired skin integrity
- Pain

Prognosis
- Overall survival depends on histology of underlying disease
- In general, 30% of the patients alive after 1 year; only 10% after 2–3 years

Syndrome of Inappropriate Antidiuretic Hormone Secretion

Epidemiology

- Can be caused by inappropriate secretion of antidiuretic hormone (ADH) of central origin or ectopic production of ADH by the tumor
- Can be caused by drugs that affect water metabolism
- Occurs in 1–2% of cancer patients

Etiology/Risk Factors

- Cancers
  - Acute leukemia
  - Bladder
  - Brain
  - Carcinoid tumors
  - Chronic leukemia
  - Duodenal
  - Esophageal
  - Ewing's sarcoma
  - Hodgkin's disease
  - Lymphosarcoma
  - Pancreatic
  - Prostate
  - Small cell lung
  - Thymoma
- Chemotherapeutic Agents
  - Cisplatin
  - Cyclophosphamide
  - Melphalan (high dose)
  - Vinblastine
  - Vincristine
- Other pharmacologic agents
  - Acetaminophen
  - Barbiturates
  - Carbamazepine
  - Chlorpropamide
  - Clofibrate
  - Histamine
  - Isoproterenol
  - Nicotine
  - Opioids
  - Thiazides
  - Thioridazine
  - Tolbutamide

Signs and Symptoms

- Mild symptoms
  - Anorexia
  - Disorientation
  - Headache
  - Mental confusion
  - Muscle cramps
  - Sleepiness
  - Weakness
  - Weight gain
- Moderate symptoms
  - Abdominal cramps
  - Diarrhea
  - Hostility/irritability
  - Lethargy
  - Nausea and vomiting
  - Oliguria
  - Personality changes
  - Sluggish DTRs
  - Weakness
- Severe symptoms
  - Coma
  - Death
  - Seizures

Diagnostic Tests

- BUN and creatinine
- Neurologic examination
- Radioimmunoassay of serum PTH
- Serum calcium level
- Serum osmolality
- Serum potassium level
- Serum sodium level
- Urine osmolality
- Urine sodium level

D

Treatment

- Eliminate underlying cause
- Fluid restriction: for serum sodium between 125 and 134 mEq/L decrease fluids to 800–1000 ml/day; for serum sodium < 120 mEq/L, decrease fluids to 500 ml/day
- Demeclocycline: administer 1200 mg initially, then decrease dose to the lowest effective dose, usually between 300 and 900 mg/day
- Lithium carbonate: has been used to treat SIADH (900–1200 mg/day) but not as effective as demeclocycline
- Hypertonic saline: used for severe hyponatremia (< 115 mEq/L) associated with confusion, seizures, and muscle twitching

Patient Problems

- Confusion
- High risk for injury
- Hypervolemia

Prognosis

- Variable, depending on the underlying cause of the syndrome

Third-Space Syndrome

Epidemiology

- Shift in fluid from the vascular to the interstitial space

Etiology/Risk Factors

- Liver disease
- Major surgery with lymph node dissection (e.g., abdominoperineal resection)
- Malnutrition
- Metastatic disease in lymph nodes

Signs and Symptoms

- Loss phase
  - Hypotension
  - Increased urine specific gravity
  - Oliguria
  - Tachycardia
- Reabsorption phase
  - Hypertension
  - Increased urine output
  - Jugular venous distension
  - Rales
  - Tachycardia
  - Weight gain

Diagnostic Tests

- BUN and creatinine
- Serum electrolytes
- Urine specific gravity
- Weight

Treatment

- Loss phase
  - Maintain fluid intake-output ratio at 3:1
  - Administer plasma proteins
- Reabsorption phase
  - Decrease IV fluid rate as soon as urine output exceeds 200 ml/hour

Patient Problems

- Hypervolemia
- Hypovolemia

Prognosis

- Excellent with aggressive fluid management

Tumor Lysis Syndrome

Epidemiology

- Characterized by hyperuricemia, hyperkalemia, hyperphosphatemia, and hypocalcemia
- Occurs in patients receiving treatment for tumors with rapid growth rate and rapid cell turnover

Etiology/Risk Factors

- ALL
- Burkitt's lymphoma
- Head and neck
- Lymphosarcoma
- Metastatic medulloblastoma
- Multiple myeloma
- NHL
- Specific chemotherapeutic agents (i.e., amsacrine, homoharringtonine, etoposide, IFN-α, tamoxifen)
- T-cell lymphoma

Signs and Symptoms

- Anorexia
- Confusion
- Decreased urine output
- Diarrhea
- ECG changes (wide to absent T wave; depressed ST segment; peaked T wave; prolonged QT interval)
- Hypotension
- Impaired memory
- Irritability
- Nausea
- Paresthesias
- Positive Chvostek's sign
- Positive Trousseau's sign
- Restlessness
- Seizures
- Slurred speech
- Spastic to flaccid paralysis
- Tetany

Diagnostic Tests

- BUN and creatinine
- ECG
- Neurologic examination
- Serum calcium level
- Serum phosphate level
- Serum potassium level
- Serum uric acid level
- Urinalysis
- Urinary pH

Treatment

- Administer IV hydration (3 L/m^2 for 24–48 hours before and during chemotherapy)
- Administer allopurinol 500 mg/m^2/day; may reduce to 200 mg/m^2/day 3 days after beginning chemotherapy
- Administer sodium bicarbonate (50 mEq/L to maintain urinary pH $\geq$ 7 if patient is hyperuricemic)
- Monitor laboratory values (i.e., serum electrolytes, BUN, creatinine, uric acid, calcium, phosphorus) every 6–12 hours
- Monitor for complications: acute renal failure, congestive heart failure
- In late stages hemodialysis may be necessary

Patient Problems

- Confusion
- Congestive heart failure
- High risk for injury
- Hypervolemia
- Renal failure

Prognosis

- Uric acid stones develop in < 10% of patients
- Majority of patients treated with aggressive therapy regain normal renal function within a few days of treatment

Bibliography

Disseminated Intravascular Coagulation

Bell, T. N. (1993). Disseminated intravascular coagulation: Clinical complexities of aberrant coagulation. *Critical Care Nursing Clinics of North America, 5*(3), 389–410.

Bick, R. L. (1992). Coagulation abnormalities in malignancy: A review. *Seminars in Thrombosis and Hemostasis, 18*(4), 353–372.

Esmon, C. T. (1994). Possible involvement of cytokines in diffuse intravascular coagulation and thrombosis. *Baillieres Clinical Haematology, 7*(3), 453–468.

Glassman, A. B., & Jones, E. (1994). Thrombosis and coagulation abnormalities associated with cancer. *Annals of Clinical and Laboratory Science, 24*(1), 1–5.

Risberg, B., Andreasson, S., & Eriksson, E. (1991). Disseminated intravascular coagulation. *Acta Anaesthesiologica Scandinavica, Supplementum, 95,* 60–71.

Ectopic ACTH Production

Cederna, P., Eckhauser, F. E., & Kealey, G. P. (1993). Cushing's syndrome secondary to bronchial carcinoid secretion of ACTH: A review. *American Surgeon, 59*(7), 438–442.

Collichio, F. A., Woolf, P. D., & Brower, M. (1994). Management of patients with small cell carcinoma and the syndrome of ectopic corticotropin secretion. *Cancer, 73*(5), 1361–1367.

Winquist, E. W., Laskey, J., Crump, M., Khamsi, F., & Shepherd, F. A. (1995). Ketoconazole in the management of paraneoplastic Cushing's syndrome secondary to ectopic adrenocorticotropin production. *Journal of Clinical Oncology, 13*(1), 157–164.

Graft-versus-Host Disease: Acute

Kelemen, E., Szebeni, J., & Petranyi, G. G. (1993). Graft-versus-host disease in bone marrow transplantation: Experimental, laboratory, and clinical contributions of the last few years. *International Archives of Allergy and Immunology, 102*(4), 309–320.

Schiller, G. J., & Gale R. P. (1992). A critical reappraisal of gastrointestinal complications of allogeneic bone marrow transplantation. *Cell Transplantation, 1*(2–3), 265–269.

Tanaka, K., Sullivan, K. M., Shulman, H. M., Sale, G. E., & Tanaka, A. (1991). A clinical review: Cutaneous manifestations of acute and chronic graft-versus-host disease following bone marrow transplantation. *Journal of Dermatology, 18*(1), 11–17.

Wojno, K. J., Vogelsang, G. B., Beschorner, W. E., & Santos, G. W. (1994). Pulmonary hemorrhage as a cause of death in allogeneic bone marrow recipients with severe acute graft-versus-host disease. *Transplantation, 57*(1), 88–92.

Graft-versus-Host Disease: Chronic

Kelemen, E., Szebeni, J., & Petranyi, G. G. (1993). Graft-versus-host disease in bone marrow transplantation: Experimental, laboratory, and clinical contributions of the last few years. *International Archives of Allergy and Immunology, 102*(4), 309–320.

Siadak, M. F., Kopecky, K., & Sullivan, K. M. (1994). Reduction in transplant-related complications in patients given intravenous immunoglobulin after allogeneic marrow transplantation. *Clinical and Experimental Immunology, 97*(Suppl. 1), 53–57.

Tanaka, K., Sullivan, K. M., Shulman, H. M., Sale, G. E., & Tanaka, A. (1991). A clinical review: Cutaneous manifestations of acute and chronic graft-versus-host disease following bone marrow transplantation. *Journal of Dermatology, 18*(1), 11–17.

Hypercalcemia

Bilezikian, J. P. (1993). Clinical review 51: Management of hypercalcemia. *Journal of Clinical Endocrinology and Metabolism, 77*(6), 1445–1449.

Ikeda, K., & Ogata, E. (1995). Humoral hypercalcemia of malignancy: Some enigmas on the clinical features. *Journal of Cellular Biochemistry, 57*(3), 384–391.

Kaplan, M. (1994). Hypercalcemia of malignancy: A review of advances in pathophysiology. *Oncology Nursing Forum, 21*(6), 1039–1046.

Kinirons, M. T. (1993). Newer agents for the treatment of malignant hypercalcemia. *American Journal of the Medical Sciences, 305*(6), 403–406.

Intestinal Obstruction

Fainsinger, R. L., Spachynski, K., Hanson, J., & Bruera, E. (1994). Symptom control in terminally ill patients with malignant bowel obstruction (MBO). *Journal of Pain and Symptom Management, 9*(1), 12–18.

Landercasper, J., Cogbill, T. H., Merry, W. H., Stolee, R. T., & Strutt, P. J. (1993). Long-term outcome after hospitalization for small-bowel obstruction. *Archives of Surgery, 128*(7), 765–770.

Lau, P. W., & Lorentz, T. G. (1993). Results of surgery for malignant bowel obstruction in advanced, unresectable, recurrent colorectal cancer. *Diseases of the Colon and Rectum, 36*(1), 61–64.

Ripamonti, C. (1994). Management of bowel obstruction in advanced cancer. *Current Opinion in Oncology, 6*(4), 351–357.

Ripamonti, C. (1994). Management of bowel obstruction in advanced cancer patients. *Journal of Pain and Symptom Management, 9*(3), 193–200.

Ripamonti, C., De Conno, F., Ventafridda, V., Rossi, B., & Baines, M. J. (1993). Management of bowel obstruction in advanced and terminal cancer patients. *Annals of Oncology, 4*(1), 15–21.

Wiseman, L. R., & Faulds, D. (1994). Cisapride. An updated review of its pharmacology and therapeutic efficacy as a prokinetic agent in gastrointestinal motility disorders. *Drugs, 47*(1), 116–152.

Intracranial Hemorrhage

Diringer, M. N. (1993). Intracerebral hemorrhage: Pathophysiology and management. *Critical Care Medicine, 21*(10), 1591–1603.

Lilleyman, J. S. (1994). Intracranial haemorrhage in idiopathic thrombocytopenic purpura. Paediatric Haematology Forum of the British Society for Haematology. *Archives of Disease in Childhood, 71*(3), 251–253.

Meyer, F. B., Morita, A., Puumala, M. R., & Nichols, D. A. (1995). Medical and surgical management of intracranial aneurysms. *Mayo Clinic Proceedings, 70*(2), 153–172.

Weaver, J. P., & Fisher, M. (1994). Subarachnoid hemorrhage: An update of pathogenesis, diagnosis and management. *Journal of the Neurological Sciences, 125*(2), 119–131.

Neoplastic Cardiac Tamponade

Olson, J. E., Ryan, M. B., & Blumenstock, D. A. (1995). Eleven years' experience with pericardial-peritoneal window in the management of malignant and benign pericardial effusions. *Annals of Surgical Oncology, 2*(2), 165–169.

Pleural Effusion

Andrews, C. O., & Gora, M. L. (1994). Pleural effusions: Pathophysiology and management. *Annals of Pharmacotherapy, 28*(7–8), 894–903.

Boggs, D. S., & Kinasewitz, G. T. (1995). Review: Pathophysiology of the pleural space. *American Journal of the Medical Sciences, 309*(1), 53–59.

Gebbia, N., Mannino, R., Di Dino, A., Maxhouni, L., Bellone, N., Cinque, L., Liuzza, A., La Motta, P., Cannata, G., & Gulotta, G. (1994). Intracavitary treatment of malignant pleural and peritoneal effusions in cancer patients. *Anticancer Research, 14*(2B), 739–745.

D

Moffett, M. J., & Ruckdeschel, J. C. (1992). Bleomycin and tetracycline in malignant pleural effusions: A review. *Seminars in Oncology, 19*(2, Suppl. 5), 59–62; discussion 62–63.

Pneumocystis carinii Pneumonia

Bennett, C. L., Horner, R. D., Weinstein, R. A., Dickinson, G. M., DeHovitz, J. A., Cohn, S. E., Kessler, H. A., Jacobson, J., Goetz, M. B., & Simberkoff, M. (1995). Racial differences in care among hospitalized patients with *Pneumocystis carinii* pneumonia in Chicago, New York, Los Angeles, Miami, and Raleigh-Durham. *Archives of Internal Medicine, 155*(15), 1586–1592.

Gallant, J. E., McAvinue, S. M., Moore, R. D., Bartlett, J. G., Stanton, D. L., & Chaisson, R. E. (1995). The impact of prophylaxis on outcome and resource utilization in *Pneumocystis carinii* pneumonia. *Chest, 107*(4), 1018–1023.

Martin, M. A., Cox, P. H., Beck, K., Styer, C. M., & Beall, G. N. (1992). A comparison of the effectiveness of three regimens in the prevention of *Pneumocystis carinii* pneumonia in human immunodeficiency virus–infected patients. *Archives of Internal Medicine, 152*(3), 523–528.

Sepkowitz, K. A. (1993). *Pneumocystis carinii* pneumonia in patients without AIDS. *Clinical Infectious Diseases, 17*(Suppl. 2), S416–S422.

Sepkowitz, K. A. (1992). *Pneumocystis carinii* pneumonia among patients with neoplastic disease. *Seminars in Respiratory Infections, 7*(2), 114–121.

Septic Shock

Bone, R. C. (1993). Gram-negative sepsis: A dilemma of modern medicine. *Clinical Microbiology Reviews, 6*(1), 57–68.

Bone, R. C. (1994). Sepsis and its complications: The clinical problem. *Critical Care Medicine, 22*(7), S8–S11.

Burrell, R. (1994). Human responses to bacterial endotoxin. *Circulatory Shock, 43*(3), 137–153.

Hazinski, M. F., Iberti, T. J., MacIntyre, N. R., Parker, M. M., Tribett, D., Prion, S., & Chmel, H. (1993). Epidemiology, pathophysiology and clinical presentation of gram-negative sepsis. *American Journal of Critical Care, 2*(3), 224–235.

Kokiko, J. (1993). Septic shock: A review and update for the emergency department clinician. *Journal of Emergency Nursing, 19*(2), 102–108.

Lynn, W. A., & Cohen, J. (1995). Adjunctive therapy for septic shock: A review of experimental approaches. *Clinical Infectious Diseases, 20*(1), 143–158.

Natanson, C., Hoffman, W. D., Suffredini, A. F., Eichacker, P. Q., & Danner, R. L. (1994). Selected treatment strategies for septic shock based on proposed mechanisms of pathogenesis. *Annals of Internal Medicine, 120*(9), 771–783.

Suffredini, A. F. (1994). Current prospects for the treatment of clinical sepsis. *Critical Care Medicine, 22*(7), S12–S18.

Spinal Cord Compression

Hill, M. E., Richards, M. A., Gregory, W. M., Smith, P., & Rubens, R. D. (1993). Spinal cord compression in breast cancer: A review of 70 cases. *British Journal of Cancer, 68*(5), 969–973.

Jordan, J. E., Donaldson, S. S., & Enzmann, D. R. (1995). Cost effectiveness and outcome assessment of magnetic resonance imaging in diagnosing cord compression. *Cancer, 75*(10), 2579–2586.

Podd, T. J., Carpenter, D. S., Baughan, C. A., Percival, D., & Dyson, P. (1992). Spinal cord compression: Prognosis and implications for treatment fractionation. *Clinical Oncology (Royal College of Radiologists), 4*(6), 341–344.

Superior Vena Cava Syndrome

de Mayolo, J. A., Sridhar, K. S., Kunhardt, B., & Rao, R. K. (1992). Superior vena cava obstruction in a patient with chronic lymphocytic leukemia and lung cancer. *American Journal of Clinical Oncology, 15*(4), 352–355.

Yellin, A., Rosen, A., Reichert, N., & Lieberman, Y. (1990). Superior vena cava syndrome. The myth—the facts. *American Review of Respiratory Disease, 141*(5, Pt. 1), 1114–1118.

Syndrome of Inappropriate Antidiuretic Hormone Secretion

Talmi, Y. P., Hoffman, H. T., & McCabe, B. F. (1992). Syndrome of inappropriate secretion of arginine vasopressin in patients with cancer of the head and neck. *Annals of Otology, Rhinology and Laryngology, 101*(11), 946–949.

Tumor Lysis Syndrome

Drakos, P., Bar-Ziv, J., & Catane, R. (1994). Tumor lysis syndrome in nonhematologic malignancies. Report of a case and review of the literature. *American Journal of Clinical Oncology, 17*(6), 502–505.

Fleming, D. R., & Doukas, M. A. (1992). Acute tumor lysis syndrome in hematologic malignancies. *Leukemia and Lymphoma, 8*(4–5), 315–318.

Veenstra, J., Krediet, R. T., Somers, R., & Arisz, L. (1994). Tumour lysis syndrome and acute renal failure in Burkitt's lymphoma. Description of 2 cases and a review of the literature on prevention and management. *Netherlands Journal of Medicine, 45*(5), 211–216.

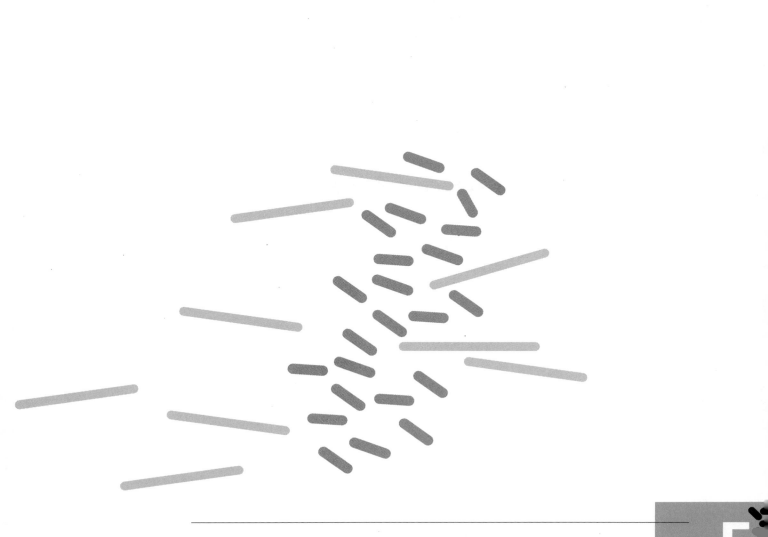

AIDS-Related Conditions

E

Aspergillus Infection

Epidemiology

- Rare complication of AIDS
- Usually seen in patients with advanced disease
- Most patients present with pulmonary disease

Signs and Symptoms

- Cough
- Elevated serum LDH
- Fever
- Pleuritic chest pain

Diagnostic Tests

- Blood cultures
- Chest radiography
- Tissue biopsy

Treatment

- Amphotericin B: 0.8–1.0 mg/kg/day IV; decrease to 0.6 mg/kg/day after week 1 and continue until total dose of at least 2 g is administered
- Itraconazole: 200–400 mg/day

Potential Problems

- Anxiety
- Fatigue
- Fever
- Impaired gas exchange
- Pain

Adverse Effects from Treatment

- Amphotericin B: decreased renal function, hypokalemia, thrombocytopenia, flushing, generalized pain, seizures, chills, fever, phlebitis, headache, anemia, anorexia
- Itraconazole: nausea, vomiting, rash

Candidiasis

Epidemiology

- Fungal infection
- Often the first opportunistic infection
- Common sites: oral cavity, esophagus, vagina, rectum, skin

Signs and Symptoms

- Oral
  - Burning sensation
  - Inflamed or atrophic mucosa
  - Oral discomfort
  - Taste changes
  - Whitish, furry, or cheesy exudate
- Esophagus
  - Chest pain
  - Dysphagia
  - Odynophagia

Diagnostic Tests

- KOH preparation (oral)
- Endoscopy with biopsy (esophageal)
- Barium swallow (esophageal)

Treatment

- Oral: nystatin suspension (400,000–600,000 units q.i.d.), nystatin pastille (1–2 pastilles q.i.d.), clotrimazole troche (10 mg 5 times/day), ketoconazole (200 mg/day PO), fluconazole (50–100 mg/day PO), itraconazole (100 mg/day PO), amphotericin B (0.3–0.5 mg/kg/day IV); average duration of therapy 7–14 days
- Esophageal: ketoconazole (400–600 mg/day PO), fluconazole (200–400 mg/day PO), itraconazole (200–400 mg/day PO)

Potential Problems

- Decreased nutritional intake
- Dysphagia
- Fever
- Pain
- Taste changes

Adverse Effects of Treatment

- Ketoconazole: nausea, vomiting, anorexia, headache, epigastric pain, photophobia, thrombocytopenia, elevated transaminases
- Clotrimazole: abnormal liver function tests, nausea, vomiting
- Fluconazole: nausea, headache, skin rash, vomiting, abdominal pain, diarrhea, elevated transaminases
- Itraconazole: nausea, vomiting, edema, rash, headache, hypokalemia, hypertension, hepatitis

CNS Lymphoma

Epidemiology

- One of the first malignancies associated with HIV
- Usually undifferentiated lymphoma
- High frequency of extranodal involvement
- Poor prognosis

Signs and Symptoms

- Aphasia
- Confusion
- Cranial nerve palsy
- Headache
- Hemiparesis
- Lethargy
- Memory loss
- Seizures

Diagnostic Tests

- Brain biopsy
- CSF cytology
- CT
- MRI

Treatment

- Radiation therapy: usually whole-brain irradiation with 4000–5000 cGy over 3 weeks

Potential Problems

- Anxiety
- Confusion
- Fatigue
- Impaired cognition
- Impaired physical mobility
- Impaired verbal communication
- Pain
- Potential for injury

Adverse Effects of Treatment

- Radiation therapy: change in mental status, impaired cognitive functioning

Coccidioidomycosis

Epidemiology
- Fungal disease caused by *Coccidioides immitis*
- Organism endemic in Southwestern United States
- Lungs are primary site of infection
- Extrapulmonary sites include: skin, meninges, lymph nodes, liver

Signs and Symptoms
- Cough
- Fatigue
- Fever
- Malaise
- Pleuritic chest pain
- Weight loss

Diagnostic Tests
- Bronchoscopy
- Culture
- IgM and IgG tests

Treatment
- Definitive treatment is unknown
- Amphotericin B: 0.5–1.0 mg/kg IV daily; with improvement, reduce dose to 50 mg 3 times a week until a total dose of 1.0–2.0 g is reached
- Fluconazole: 400 mg PO, daily follows IV amphotericin B therapy

Potential Problems
- Anxiety
- Fatigue
- Impaired gas exchange
- Ineffective breathing pattern
- Pain

Adverse Effects of Treatment
- Amphotericin B: decreased renal function, hypokalemia, thrombocytopenia, flushing, pain, seizures, chills, fever, phlebitis, headache, anemia, anorexia
- Fluconazole: nausea, headache, skin rash, abdominal pain, vomiting, diarrhea, elevated transaminases

Cryptococcal Meningitis

Epidemiology

- *Cryptococcus neoformans* is causative organism
- Fungal infection that has a marked predilection for the brain and meninges
- Ubiquitous fungus in the soil
- Accounts for 5–8% of all opportunistic infections in AIDS patients

Signs and Symptoms

- Behavior changes
- Fatigue
- Fever
- Headache
- Memory loss
- Meningismus
- Mental status changes
- Nausea and vomiting
- Papilledema
- Photophobia
- Seizures

Diagnostic Tests

- Brain CT
- Lumbar puncture
  - CSF cryptococcal antigen
  - Cell count
  - Fungal culture
  - Glucose level
  - India ink preparation for fungi
  - Protein level
  - Opening pressure
- MRI
- Serum cryptococcal antigen

Treatment

- Amphotericin B: 0.4–0.6 mg/kg/day IV for at least 6 weeks or 0.5–1.0 mg/kg/day IV, with or without flucytosine 100 mg/kg/day IV, q6h for 2–3 weeks
- Fluconazole: 400 mg/day PO, for 8–12 weeks

Potential Problems

- Anxiety
- Confusion
- Fatigue
- Pain
- Potential for injury

Adverse Effects of Treatment

- Amphotericin B: decreased renal function, hypokalemia, thrombocytopenia, flushing, generalized pain, seizures, chills, fever, phlebitis, headache, anemia, anorexia
- Fluconazole: nausea, headache, skin rash, vomiting, abdominal pain, diarrhea, elevated transaminases

Cryptosporidiosis

Epidemiology

- *Cryptosporidium* is a coccidian protozoan
- Intracellular parasite that usually infects cells of the intestine
- Can cause acute or chronic diarrhea

Signs and Symptoms

- Cramping abdominal pain
- Flatulence
- Malaise
- Myalgias
- Nausea
- Vomiting
- Watery diarrhea
- Weight loss

Diagnostic Tests

- Acid-fast stain of stool
- Intestinal biopsy

Treatment

- Difficult to treat
- Trial of therapy with paromonomycin 500 mg PO q.i.d. for up to 30 days
- Supportive treatment with antidiarrheal drugs and hydration

Potential Problems

- Anorexia
- Fatigue
- Fluid volume deficit
- Nutritional deficit
- Pain
- Rectal skin breakdown

Adverse Effects of Treatment

- Paromonomycin: nephrotoxicity

Cytomegalovirus Colitis

Epidemiology
- CMV may be sexually transmitted
- Herpesvirus group of double-stranded DNA viruses
- Latent virus in the general population
- Most patients who develop CMV disease have CD4 counts < 50

Signs and Symptoms
- Abdominal pain
- Diarrhea (often bloody)
- Diffuse mucosal ulceration
- Erythema
- Esophagitis
- Fever
- Gastritis
- Submucosal hemorrhage

Diagnostic Tests
- Culture virus from tissue
- Endoscopy

Treatment
- Ganciclovir 10 mg/kg/day IV b.i.d. for 14 days (induction); 5 mg/kg/day maintenance

Potential Problems
- Dysphagia
- Fluid volume deficit
- Nutritional deficit
- Pain
- Rectal skin breakdown
- Weight loss

Adverse Effects of Treatment
- Ganciclovir: myelosuppression, rash, nausea, vomiting, renal insufficiency, suppression of spermatogenesis

Cytomegalovirus Retinitis

Epidemiology

- CMV can be sexually transmitted
- Herpesvirus group of double-stranded DNA viruses
- Latent virus in the general population
- CMV is the most common cause of blindness in AIDS patients
- Most patients who develop CMV disease have CD4 counts < 50

Signs and Symptoms

- Blurred vision
- Perivascular exudate
- Retinal hemorrhages
- Scotomas
- Unilateral visual field loss

Diagnostic Tests

- Fundoscopic examination
- Classic "crumbled cheese and ketchup" appearance of exudate with heme

Treatment

- Ganciclovir 5 mg/kg, q12h IV for 14–21 days (induction), followed by 6 mg/kg daily, 5–7 days/week for life
- Foscarnet dose is adjusted based on renal function; 60 mg/kg IV q8h for 14–21 days (induction) followed by 90–120 mg/kg IV daily (maintenance)

Potential Problems

- Anxiety
- Decreased visual acuity
- Potential for injury

Adverse Effects of Treatment

- Ganciclovir: myelosuppression, rash, nausea, vomiting, renal insufficiency, suppression of spermatogenesis
- Foscarnet: renal dysfunction, renal failure, seizures, tetany, hypocalcemia, hyperphosphatemia

Herpes Simplex

Epidemiology
- Common sexually transmitted disease
- Disseminated HSV infection may be life-threatening

Signs and Symptoms
- General
  - Pain
  - Painful vesicular eruption
  - Ulcers
- Genital lesions
  - Adenopathy
  - Dysuria
  - Lesions on the genital area
- Orolabial lesions
  - Adenopathy
  - Vesicular eruptions on the lips, tongue, and oral mucosa
- Rectal lesions
  - Severe, painful, invasive lesions

Diagnostic Tests
- Previous history
- Tzanck smear
- Viral culture

Treatment
- Acyclovir: 200 mg PO, q4h, 5 times a day for 10–14 days; for frequent recurrences, give 200 mg PO t.i.d. or 400 mg PO b.i.d.

Potential Problems
- Pain

Adverse Effects of Treatment
- Acyclovir: arthralgias, diarrhea, headache, nausea, vomiting, dizziness

Herpes Zoster

Epidemiology
- Caused by reactivation of the VZV latent in dorsal root ganglia
- May be the first sign of immunocompromise

Signs and Symptoms
- Itching
- Deep, aching pain
- Erythematous rash to vesicles
- Fatigue
- Fever
- Headache
- Malaise
- Vesicular rash confined to one dermatome

Diagnostic Tests
- Direct immunofluorescence
- History
- Physical examination
- Tzanck smear
- Viral cultures

Treatment
- Acyclovir 800 mg q4h PO five times a day or 30 mg/kg/day, IV, for 7–10 days
- Pain management with opioid analgesics

Potential Problems
- Fatigue
- Pain

Adverse Effects of Treatment
- Acyclovir: arthralgias, diarrhea, headache, nausea, vomiting, dizziness
- Opioids: constipation, sedation

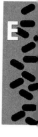

Histoplasmosis

Epidemiology
- Introduced into the body through inhalation
- Infection begins in the lungs; can become systemic
- Fungus endemic to South Central United States

Signs and Symptoms
- Adenopathy
- Anemia
- Cough
- Fever
- Hepatosplenomegaly
- Jaundice
- Leukopenia
- Malaise
- Skin lesions
- Thrombocytopenia
- Weight loss

Diagnostic Tests
- Cultures of bone marrow, blood, urine, and biopsy tissue
- Radioimmunoassay of histopolysaccharide antigen
- Serologic tests for *Histoplasma* organisms

Treatment
- Amphotericin B: 0.4–0.6 mg/kg/day IV for 10–12 weeks (induction); optimal maintenance dose and duration are unknown
- Itraconazole: 200 mg PO once or twice a day for 3 months or more; has been used as maintenance therapy

Potential Problems
- Decreased activity tolerance
- Fatigue
- Ineffective airway clearance
- Nutritional deficit
- Pain
- Potential for injury

Adverse Effects of Treatment
- Amphotericin B: decreased renal function, hypokalemia, thrombocytopenia, flushing, generalized pain, seizures, chills, fever, phlebitis, headache, anemia, anorexia
- Itraconazole: nausea, rash, vomiting

HIV-Associated Dementia

Epidemiology
- Chronic progressive CNS disorder characterized by cognitive, motor, and behavioral dysfunction
- Also called *AIDS dementia complex* (ADC)
- Most common CNS complication in patients with AIDS

Signs and Symptoms
- Behavioral: apathy, reduced spontaneity, social withdrawal
- Cognitive: poor concentration, forgetfulness, slowness
- Mental status: inattention, psychomotor slowing, impairment of processing, global dementia, mutism, organic psychosis
- Motor findings: impaired rapid movements, ataxia, tremor, hypertonia, paraparesis, incontinence, myoclonus, loss of balance, leg weakness, clumsiness

Diagnostic Tests
- CSF protein
- CT
- MRI
- Magnetic resonance spectroscopy

Treatment
- Manage symptoms
- Antiretroviral therapy: zidovudine 200 mg q4h while awake

Potential Problems
- Anxiety
- Impaired cognitive functioning
- Impaired communication pattern
- Impaired mobility
- Potential for injury
- Self-care deficit

Adverse Effects of Treatment
- Zidovudine: granulocytopenia, anemia, headache, nausea and vomiting, fatigue, myopathy

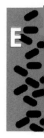

Isosporiasis

Epidemiology
- Caused by *Isospora belli,* a parasite
- More common in tropical and subtropical climates

Signs and Symptoms
- Biliary tract obstruction
- Intractable diarrhea
- Malabsorption
- Malnutrition
- Weakness
- Weight loss

Diagnostic Tests
- Stool for ova and parasites $\times$ 3
- Serum electrolytes
- Steatorrhea

Treatment
- TMP-SMX: 160/800 mg PO q.i.d. for 10 days followed by TMP-SMX 160/800 PO b.i.d. for 21 days
- For sulfa allergy: pyrimethamine 75 mg/day PO with folinic acid 10–25 mg/day PO

Potential Problems
- Abdominal pain
- Diarrhea
- Fluid volume deficit
- Perirectal skin breakdown

Adverse Effects of Treatment
- TMP-SMX: rash, fever, leukopenia, hyponatremia, abnormal liver function tests
- Pyrimethamine: megaloblastic anemia, thrombocytopenia, leukopenia, anorexia, vomiting, ataxia, tremors, increased liver enzymes, hypersensitivity reaction

Kaposi's Sarcoma

Epidemiology

- Originates in vascular or lymphatic endothelial cells
- Exact cause is unknown

Signs and Symptoms

- GI disease
  - Bleeding
  - Diarrhea
  - Dysphagia
  - Malabsorption
- Lesion on the skin or oral cavity
- Lymphatic involvement
  - Lymphadenopathy
  - Lymphedema
- Oral lesions
  - Dysphagia
  - Pain
  - Pigmented, red, purple, brown lesions
- Pulmonary disease
  - Cough
  - Dyspnea on exertion
  - Fever
  - Pleural effusion
  - Respiratory distress
  - Shortness of breath
  - Tachypnea

Diagnostic Tests

- Bronchoscopy (lungs)
- Punch biopsy (skin)

Treatment

- Treatment for local lesions: small lesions are treated only if they are painful or causing cosmetic problems
  - Modalities used include radiation therapy, cryotherapy, intralesional injections of vinblastine
- Progressive cutaneous or disseminated disease is treated with chemotherapy (e.g., vinblastine, vincristine, bleomycin, adriamycin, etoposide)
  - Liposomal encapsulated daunorubicin and adriamycin is under evaluation

Potential Problems

- Altered body image
- Diarrhea
- Impaired gas exchange
- Nutritional deficit
- Pain
- Sexual dysfunction

Adverse Effects of Treatment

- Chemotherapy: bone marrow suppression, fever, diarrhea, alopecia

Molluscum Contagiosum

Epidemiology

- Cutaneous poxvirus infection
- Usually sexually transmitted
- Incidence is approximately 10–20%

Signs and Symptoms

- Flesh-colored umbilicated papules
- Lesions are distributed along face, neck, scalp, and trunk

Diagnostic Tests

- Skin biopsy
- Visual examination

Treatment

- Curettage
- Electrocoagulation
- Liquid nitrogen and cryosurgery
- Retin-A cream 0.01% applied once a day

Potential Problem

- Body image disturbance

Adverse Effects of Treatment

- None

Mycobacterium avium Complex

Epidemiology

- Includes both *M. avium* and *M. avium-intracellulare*
- Acid-fast, slow-growing bacilli
- Occurs late in the course of HIV infection
- Occurs in approximately 50% of patients infected with HIV

Signs and Symptoms

- Abdominal pain
- Anemia
- Anorexia
- Diarrhea
- Fatigue
- Fever
- Hepatosplenomegaly
- Night sweats
- Palpable abdominal lymphadenopathy
- Weight loss

Diagnostic Tests

- Blood culture
- Bone marrow culture
- Sputum culture
- Stool culture
- Tissue culture (e.g., lymph node)

Treatment

- Combination therapy is required
- Amikacin: 7.5 mg/kg/day IV/IM for up to 8 weeks
- Azithromycin: 500–900 mg/day PO
- Ciprofloxacin: 750 mg PO b.i.d.
- Clarithromycin: 500 mg PO b.i.d. (can increase to 1000 mg b.i.d.)
- Clofazamine: 100–200 mg/day PO
- Ethambutol: 25 mg/kg/day for 6 weeks; then, 15 mg/kg/day PO (maximum 1200 mg)
- Rifampin: 300 mg/day PO
- Oral medications are continued for life

Potential Problems

- Anorexia
- Fatigue
- Nutritional deficit
- Pain
- Perirectal skin breakdown
- Potential for injury

Adverse Effects of Treatment

- Amikacin: nephrotoxicity, ototoxicity
- Azithromycin: nausea, diarrhea, abdominal pain, ototoxicity
- Ciprofloxacin: restlessness, nausea, diarrhea, vomiting, abdominal pain, rash
- Clarithromycin: headache, diarrhea, nausea, abnormal taste, ototoxicity
- Clofazamine: abdominal pain, nausea, abnormal liver enzymes, skin dryness, diarrhea, rash, itching
- Ethambutol: abnormal liver enzymes, increased uric acid levels, optic neuritis, peripheral neuritis, headache, dizziness, nausea, vomiting
- Rifampin: fever, chills, myalgias, headache, nausea, vomiting, thrombocytopenia, interstitial nephritis, abnormal liver function tests, anemia

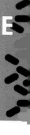

Mycobacterium tuberculosis Infection

Epidemiology

- May be first sign of immunodeficiency
- Recent reports of multidrug-resistant MTB
- Approximately 75% of patients have extrapulmonary disease (e.g., pleura, lymph nodes, bone marrow, peripheral blood, GI and GU tract, brain, bone, skin, soft tissue, pericardium)

Signs and Symptoms

- Cough
- Fever
- Hemoptysis
- Night sweats
- Weight loss

Diagnostic Tests

- Acid-fast bacilli staining and culture
- Chest radiography
- PPD

Treatment

- Combination therapy
  - Isoniazid (INH): 5–10 mg/kg/day; usually 300 mg/day PO for 6–12 months *and*
  - Pyridoxine: 50 mg/day PO for 6 months or as long as INH treatment is needed *and*
  - Rifampin: 9 mg/kg/day; usually 600 mg/day PO for 6–12 months *and*
  - Pyrazinamide: 25 mg/kg/day PO for 2 months
- For multidrug-resistant TB, up to 5 or 6 drugs are recommended, including INH, rifampin, pyrazinamide, ethambutol, an aminoglycoside, and aquinolone
- INH prophylaxis: 300 mg/day PO for 12 months for all HIV/PPD–positive persons not previously treated

Potential Problems

- Anxiety
- Discomfort
- Fever
- Impaired gas exchange
- Nutritional deficit
- Respiratory distress

Adverse Effects of Treatment

- INH: peripheral neuropathy, skin rash, hepatotoxicity
- Pyridoxine: neuropathy with high doses
- Rifampin: hepatotoxicity, diarrhea, fever
- Pyrazinamide: hepatotoxicity, fever, rash

Nocardia Infection

Epidemiology

- Gram-positive actinomycete
- Causes liquefaction, necrosis, and abscesses
- Most infections involve lung and CNS
- Can affect the abdomen

Signs and Symptoms

- Abdomen
  - Abdominal pain
  - Abdominal tenderness
  - Ascites
  - Fever
- CNS
  - Brain abscess
- Lung
  - Fever
  - Malaise
  - Night sweats
  - Productive cough
  - Weight loss

Diagnostic Tests

- Abdominal CT
- Abdominal radiography
- Chest radiography
- Culture
- Head CT

Treatment

- TMP-SMX: start with IV preparation and continue with oral preparation of one double-strength tablet b.i.d. for at least 6 months

Potential Problems

- Anxiety
- Discomfort
- Fatigue
- Nutritional deficit

Adverse Effects of Treatment

- TMP-SMX: fever, rash, leukopenia, hyponatremia, elevated liver function tests

Non-Hodgkin's Lymphoma

Epidemiology
- High-grade B-cell NHL
- Occurs in 3% of patients with HIV disease

Signs and Symptoms
- Anorectal abscess
- Fever
- Lymphadenopathy
- Night sweats
- Weight loss

Diagnostic Test
- Biopsy

Treatment
- No successful treatment has been established for NHL in AIDS patients
- Combination chemotherapy includes methotrexate, bleomycin, doxorubicin, cyclophosphamide, vincristine, and dexamethasone (modified m-BACQD regimen)
- Newer combination therapy includes chemotherapy, antiretroviral agents, prophylaxis for PCP, and colony-stimulating factors

Potential Problems
- Fatigue
- Nutritional deficit
- Pain
- Perirectal skin breakdown

Adverse Effects of Treatment
- Variable, depending on the treatment regimen

Pneumocystis carinii Pneumonia

Epidemiology
- Protozoan or fungus
- Most common opportunistic infection in patients with HIV disease
- > 65% of patients with HIV develop PCP

Signs and Symptoms
- Cough
- Cyanosis
- Diarrhea
- Dyspnea
- Fatigue
- Fever
- Malaise
- Rales
- Shortness of breath
- Tachypnea
- Weight loss
- Wheezes

Diagnostic Tests
- Arterial blood gases
- Bronchoscopy
- CD4 counts
- Chest radiography
- Gallium scan
- LDH level
- Sputum induction

Treatment

- TMP-SMX: 2 double-strength tablets, PO, q.i.d.

or

- Dapsone: 100 mg/day PO and TMP 20 mg/kg/day PO in 4 divided doses

or

- Atovaquone: 750 mg PO t.i.d.

or

- Clindamycin: 450 mg PO q.i.d. and primaquine 30 mg/day PO
- Continue treatment 14–21 days

Potential Problems
- Anxiety
- Discomfort
- Fatigue
- Impaired gas exchange
- Ineffective breathing pattern
- Nutritional deficit

Adverse Effects of Treatment
- TMP-SMX: rash, fever, leukopenia, hyponatremia, elevated liver function tests
- Dapsone: nausea, vomiting, hemolytic anemia, agranulocytosis, methemoglobinemia, peripheral neuropathy
- Atovaquone: rash, diarrhea, nausea, headache, vomiting, fever
- Clindamycin: diarrhea
- Primaquine: nausea, vomiting, hemolytic anemia, methemoglobinemia, bone marrow suppression

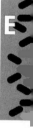

Progressive Multifocal Leukoencephalopathy

Epidemiology

- Opportunistic infection caused by the JC virus
- Probably reactivation of a latent virus
- Human papillomavirus causes selective demyelination of the white matter of the brain

Signs and Symptoms

- Abnormal gait
- Ataxia
- Cognitive dysfunction
- Dementia
- Focal neurologic deficits
- Headache
- Hemiparesis
- Sensory deficits
- Spastic hemiparesis
- Speech disturbances
- Visual deficits
- Visual field loss
- Weakness

Diagnostic Tests

- Brain biopsy
- CT
- MRI

Treatment

- No proven therapy for PML

Potential Problems

- Alteration in skin integrity
- Decreased mobility
- Impaired cognitive function
- Inability to communicate
- Pain
- Potential for injury
- Self-care deficit
- Visual disturbances

Adverse Effects of Treatment

- None

Salmonellosis

Epidemiology

- *Salmonellae* are gram negative bacteria
- Incidence in patients with AIDS is 100 times greater than in the general population
- Acquired by ingestion of contaminated food, direct fecal-oral spread, transfusion of contaminated blood

Signs and Symptoms

- Anorexia
- Chills
- Diarrhea
- Fever
- Sweats
- Weight loss

Diagnostic Tests

- Blood culture
- Stool culture

Treatment

- Initial treatment: use IV therapy until symptoms improve, then switch to an oral regimen to finish a 14-day course of therapy
  - Ceftriaxone: 1–2 g IV q24h

or

  - TMP-SMX: 5–15 mg/kg, IV, in divided doses q6h

or

  - Ampicillin: 500 mg IV q6h

or

  - Chloramphenicol: 500 mg, IV, q6h

plus

  - Consider rifampin 300 mg/day PO for synergistic effect

Potential Problems

- Diarrhea
- Discomfort
- Fatigue
- Fluid volume deficit
- Nutritional deficit
- Perirectal skin breakdown

Adverse Effects of Treatment

- Ceftriaxone: nausea, vomiting, diarrhea, rashes, phlebitis
- TMP-SMX: rash, fever, leukopenia, hyponatremia, abnormal liver function tests
- Ampicillin: rashes, diarrhea
- Chloramphenicol: bone marrow depression
- Rifampin: nausea, vomiting, heartburn, abdominal pain, flatulence, diarrhea, red discoloration of all body fluids

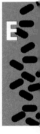

Shigellosis

Epidemiology
- *Shigella sonnei* is a causative organism in the United States

Signs and Symptoms
- Anorexia
- Bloody stool
- Chills
- Diarrhea
- Fever
- Headache
- Lower abdominal pain
- Malaise
- Tenesmus

Diagnostic Tests
- Blood culture
- Stool culture

Treatment
- TMP-SMX: one double-strength tablet PO b.i.d.

or
- Ciprofloxacin: 750 mg PO b.i.d.

Potential Problems
- Anorexia
- Fatigue
- Fluid volume deficit
- Nutritional deficit
- Pain
- Perirectal skin breakdown

Adverse Effects of Treatment
- TMP-SMX: rash, fever, leukopenia, hyponatremia, elevated liver function tests
- Ciprofloxacin: restlessness, nausea, vomiting, diarrhea, abdominal pain

Staphylococcus aureus Infection

Epidemiology

· *S. aureus* is not normal skin flora
· Abscess formation is common

Signs and Symptoms

· Boils may form
· Fasciititis
· Infection begins around hair follicles
· Myositis

Diagnostic Tests

· Blood culture
· Wound culture

Treatment

- • Drain abscess
- • Dicloxacillin: 500 mg PO q.i.d. for 7–10 days
- *or*
- • Cephalexin: 500 mg PO q.i.d. for 7–10 days

Potential Problems

· Impaired skin integrity
· Pain

Adverse Effects of Treatment

· Dicloxacillin: nausea, vomiting, rash, diarrhea, allergic reaction
· Cephalexin: nausea, vomiting, diarrhea, rash

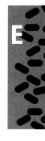

Syphilis

Epidemiology

- Coinfection with HIV is common
- Consider neurosyphilis in HIV-infected patients with neurologic disease

Signs and Symptoms

- Altered mental status
- Aortitis
- Chancre
- Encephalitis
- Facial palsy
- Fever
- Hearing loss
- Hemiparesis
- Hemiplegia
- Hepatitis
- Iritis
- Lymphadenopathy
- Meningitis
- Ocular symptoms
- Rash
- Retinitis

Diagnostic Tests

- Lumbar puncture
- Rapid plasma reagin
- Treponemal assays
- VDRL

Treatment

- Primary and secondary syphilis: 2.4 million units of benzathine penicillin IM, once a week for 3 consecutive weeks
- Syphilis of > 1 year's duration or latent syphilis or neurosyphilis: aqueous penicillin G 2–4 million U/day IV q4h for 10 days or procaine penicillin G 2.4 million U/day IM with probenecid 500 mg PO q.i.d. for 10 days
- Ceftriaxone: 1–2 g/day for 10–14 days has been studied

Potential Oncologic Emergencies

- Decreased hearing
- Decreased visual acuity
- Diarrhea
- Discomfort
- Fatigue
- Impaired cognitive functioning
- Impaired mobility
- Potential for injury

Adverse Effects of Treatment

- Benzathine penicillin: nausea, vomiting, diarrhea, epigastric distress, rash, pain at injection site
- Aqueous penicillin G: nausea, vomiting, diarrhea, epigastric distress, rash, phlebitis
- Procaine penicillin G: nausea, vomiting, diarrhea, epigastric distress, skin rash, pain at injection site
- Probenecid: headache, nausea, vomiting, diarrhea

Thrombocytopenia

Epidemiology
- May occur with HIV infection
- Megakaryocytes may be infected with the virus, resulting in decreased platelet production and decreased platelet survival time

Signs and Symptoms
- Bruising
- Ecchymosis
- Epistaxis
- Gingival bleeding
- Petechiae
- Rectal bleeding

Diagnostic Tests
- Bone marrow biopsy
- Platelet count

Treatment
- Several treatment options are available
- No therapy may be necessary
- Therapeutic options include: zidovudine, dapsone, vincristine, anabolic steroids, high-dose ascorbate (2–4 g/day), corticosteroids, splenectomy, intravenous immunoglobulin, low-dose splenic irradiation (900–1000 cGy over 1 month)

Potential Problems
- Anxiety
- Potential for injury

Adverse Effects of Treatment
- Highly dependent on the treatment used

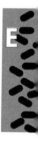

Toxoplasmosis

Epidemiology

- *Toxoplasma gondii* is a protozoan
- Cats and other animals serve as reservoirs for the organism
- Most common cause of focal encephalitis in patients with AIDS
- Transmission occurs via ingestion of contaminated food or water

Signs and Symptoms

- Abnormal gait
- Aphasia
- Chorioretinitis
- Coma
- Confusion
- Fever
- Focal neurologic deficits
- Headache
- Lethargy
- Poor condition
- Seizures
- Sensory deficits

Diagnostic Tests

- Brain biopsy
- CSF toxoplasmosis IgG antibodies
- CT
- MRI
- Serology

Treatment

- Sulfadiazine: 75 mg/kg PO loading dose, followed by 100 mg/kg/day (6–8 g) divided into 2–4 doses

with

- Pyrimethamine: 100 mg/day PO for 2 days as a loading dose, followed by 50–100 mg/day

with

- Folinic acid: 10–20 mg/day PO
- Continue treatment 6–9 weeks
- For sulfa allergy, use clindamycin 600 mg IV or PO q6h

Potential Problems

- Decreased cognitive functioning
- Decreased mobility
- Pain
- Potential for injury
- Self-care deficit

Adverse Effects of Treatment

- Sulfadiazine: renal insufficiency, hemolytic anemia, agranulocytosis, aplastic anemia, thrombocytopenia, eosinophilia, skin rash, hepatotoxicity
- Pyrimethamine: myelosuppression, megaloblastic anemia, skin rash
- Clindamycin: diarrhea

Bibliography

Aspergillosis

Duthie, R., & Denning, D. W. (1995). *Aspergillus fungemia:* Report of two cases and review. *Clinical Infectious Diseases, 20*(3), 598–605.

Keating, J. J., Rogers, T., Petrou, M., Cartledge, J. D., Woodrow, D., Nelson, M., Hawkins, D. A., & Gazzard, B. G. (1994). Management of pulmonary aspergillosis in AIDS: An emerging clinical problem. *Journal of Clinical Pathology, 47*(9), 805–809.

Khoo, S. H., & Denning, D. W. (1994). Invasive aspergillosis in patients with AIDS. *Clinical Infectious Diseases, 19*(Suppl. 1), S41–S48.

Staples, C. A., Kang, E. Y., Wright, J. L., Phillips, P., & Muller, N. L. (1995). Invasive pulmonary aspergillosis in AIDS: Radiographic, CT, and pathologic findings. *Radiology, 196*(2), 409–414.

Candidiasis

Greenspan, D., & Greenspan, J. S. (1991). Management of the oral lesions of HIV infection. *Journal of the American Dental Association, 122*(9), 26–32.

McCarthy, G. M. (1992). Host factors associated with HIV-related oral candidiasis. A review. *Oral Surgery, Oral Medicine, Oral Pathology, 73*(2), 181–186.

Reents, S., Goodwin, S. D., & Singh, V. (1993). Antifungal prophylaxis in immunocompromised hosts. *Annals of Pharmacotherapy, 27*(1), 53–60.

Sciubba, J. J. (1992). Recognizing the oral manifestations of AIDS. *Oncology, 6*(9), 64–70.

Scully, C., el-Kabir, M., & Samaranayake, L. P. (1994). *Candida* and oral candidosis: A review. *Critical Reviews in Oral Biology and Medicine, 5*(2), 125–157.

Central Nervous System Lymphoma

Dina, T. S. (1991). Primary central nervous system lymphoma versus toxoplasmosis in AIDS. *Radiology, 179*(3), 823–828.

Remick, S. C., Diamond, C., Migliozzi, J. A., Solis, O., Wagner, H., Jr., Haase, R. F., & Ruckdeschel, J. C. (1990). Primary central nervous system lymphoma in patients with and without the acquired immune deficiency syndrome. A retrospective analysis and review of the literature. *Medicine, 69*(6), 345–360.

Coccidioidomycosis

Graybill, J. R. (1993). Treatment of coccidioidomycosis. *Current Topics in Medical Mycology, 5,* 151–179.

Wheat, J. (1994). Histoplasmosis and coccidioidomycosis in individuals with AIDS. A clinical review. *Infectious Disease Clinics of North America, 8*(2), 467–482.

Wheat, J. (1995). Endemic mycoses in AIDS: A clinical review. *Clinical Microbiology Reviews, 8*(1), 146–159.

Cryptococcal Meningitis

Mitchell, D. H., Sorrell, T. C., Allworth, A. M., Heath, C. H., McGregor, A. R., Papanaoum, K., Richards, M. J., & Gottlieb, T. (1995). Cryptococcal disease of the CNS in immunocompetent hosts: Influence of cryptococcal variety on clinical manifestations and outcome. *Clinical Infectious Diseases, 20*(3), 611–616.

Nelson, M. R., Fisher, M., Cartledge, J., Rogers, T., & Gazzard, B. G. (1994). The role of azoles in the treatment and prophylaxis of cryptococcal disease in HIV infection. *AIDS, 8*(5), 651–654.

Powderly, W. G. (1993). Cryptococcal meningitis and AIDS. *Clinical Infectious Diseases, 17*(5), 837–842.

Cryptosporidiosis

Moss, P. J., Read, R. C., Kudesia, G., & McKendrick, M. W. (1995). Prolonged cryptosporidiosis during primary HIV infection. *Journal of Infection, 30*(1), 51–53.

Cytomegalovirus Colitis

Dieterich, D. T., & Rahmin, M. (1991). Cytomegalovirus colitis in AIDS: Presentation in 44 patients and a review of the literature. *Journal of Acquired Immune Deficiency Syndromes, 4*(Suppl. 1), S29–S35.

Cytomegalovirus Retinitis

Fanning, M. M., Rad, S. E., Benson, M., Vas, S., Rachlis, A., Kozousek, V., Mortimer, C., Harvey, P., Schwartz, C., & Chew, E. (1990). Foscarnet therapy of cytomegalovirus retinitis in AIDS. *Journal of Acquired Immune Deficiency Syndromes, 3*(5), 472–479.

Smith, M. A., & Brennessel, D. J. (1994). Cytomegalovirus. *Infectious Disease Clinics of North America, 8*(2), 427–438.

Dementia

Everall, I., Luthert, P., & Lantos, P. (1993). A review of neuronal damage in human immunodeficiency virus infection: Its assessment, possible mechanism and relationship to dementia. *Journal of Neuropathology and Experimental Neurology, 52*(6), 561–566.

Lipton, S. A. (1994). AIDS-related dementia and calcium homeostasis. *Annals of the New York Academy of Sciences, 747,*205–224.

Portegies, P. (1994). AIDS dementia complex: A review. *Journal of Acquired Immune Deficiency Syndromes, 7*(Suppl. 2), S38–S48.

Portegies, P. (1995). Review of antiretroviral therapy in the prevention of HIV-related AIDS dementia complex (ADC). *Drugs, 49*(Suppl. 1), 25–31.

Herpes Simplex

Becker, Y. (1990). Concepts and trends in antiviral chemotherapy in the period of AIDS: A review. *Journal of Chemotherapy, 2*(2), 91–99.

Fletcher, C. V. (1992). Treatment of herpes virus infections in HIV-infected individuals. *Annals of Pharmacotherapy, 26*(7–8), 955–962.

Herpes Zoster

Grossman, M. C., & Grossman, M. E. (1993). Chronic hyperkeratotic herpes zoster and human immunodeficiency virus infection. *Journal of the American Academy of Dermatology, 28*(2 Pt. 2), 306–308.

Histoplasmosis

Drew, R. H. (1993). Pharmacotherapy of disseminated histoplasmosis in patients with AIDS. *Annals of Pharmacotherapy, 27*(12), 1510–1518.

Wheat, J. (1994). Histoplasmosis and coccidioidomycosis in individuals with AIDS. A clinical review. *Infectious Disease Clinics of North America, 8*(2), 467–482.

Wheat, L. J., Connolly-Stringfield, P. A., Baker, R. L., Curfman, M. F., Eads, M. E., Israel, K. S., Norris, S. A., Webb, D. H., & Zeckel, M. L. (1990). Disseminated histoplasmosis in the acquired immune deficiency syndrome: Clinical findings, diagnosis and treatment, and review of the literature. *Medicine, 69*(6), 361–374.

Kaposi's Sarcoma

Aboulafia, D. M. (1994). Human immunodeficiency virus–associated neoplasms: Epidemiology, pathogenesis, and review of current therapy. *Cancer Practice, 2*(4), 297–306.

Mitsuyasu, R. T. (1993). Clinical aspects of AIDS-related Kaposi's sarcoma. *Current Opinion in Oncology, 5*(5) 835–844.

Stein, M., Spencer, D., Kuten, A., & Bezwoda, W. (1994). AIDS-related Kaposi's sarcoma: A

review. *Israel Journal of Medical Sciences,*
30(4), 298–305.

Molluscum Contagiosum

Epstein, W. L. (1992). Molluscum contagiosum.
Seminars in Dermatology, 11(3), 184–189.
Schwartz, J. J., & Myskowski, P. L. (1992).
Molluscum contagiosum in patients with human
immunodeficiency virus infection. A review of
twenty-seven patients. *Journal of the American
Academy of Dermatology, 27*(4), 583–588.

Mycobacterium avium Complex

Benson, C. A., & Ellner, J. J. (1993).
Mycobacterium avium complex infection and
AIDS: Advances in theory and practice. *Clinical
Infectious Diseases, 17*(1), 7–20.
Kissinger, P., Clark, R., Morse, A., & Brandon, W.
(1995). Comparison of multiple drug therapy
regimens for HIV-related disseminated
Mycobacterium avium complex disease. *Journal
of Acquired Immune Deficiency Syndromes and
Human Retrovirology, 9*(2), 133–137.

Mycobacterium tuberculosis

Alwood, K., Keruly, J., Moore-Rice, K., Stanton,
D. L., Chaulk, C. P., & Chaisson R. E. (1994).
Effectiveness of supervised, intermittent therapy
for tuberculosis in HIV-infected patients. *AIDS,
8*(8), 1103–1108.
Mundy, L. M., Lynch, M. M., Crowley, B. D.,
Kelly, G., Desmond, N. M., & Mulcahy, F. M.
(1994). Concomitant HIV and mycobacterial
infection in Ireland, 1987–92. *International
Journal of STD and AIDS, 5*(6), 436–441.

Nocardia

Boiron, P., Provost, F., Chevrier, G., & Dupont, B.
(1992). Review of nocardial infections in France
1987 to 1990. *European Journal of Clinical
Microbiology and Infectious Diseases, 11*(8),
709–714.

Kim, J., Minamoto, G. Y., & Grieco, M. H. (1991).
Nocardial infection as a complication of AIDS:
Report of six cases and review. *Reviews of
Infectious Diseases, 13*(4), 624–629.
McNeil, M. M., & Brown, J. M. (1994). The
medically important aerobic actinomycetes:
Epidemiology and microbiology. *Clinical
Microbiology Reviews, 7*(3), 357–417.

Progressive Multifocal Leukoencephalopathy

von Einsiedel, R. W., Fife, T. D., Aksamit, A. J.,
Cornford, M. E., Secor, D. L., Tomiyasu, U.,
Itabashi, H. H., & Vinters, H. V. (1993).
Progressive multifocal leukoencephalopathy in
AIDS: A clinicopathologic study and review of
the literature. *Journal of Neurology, 240*(7),
391–406.

Salmonella

Fish, D. N., & Danziger, L. H. (1993). Neglected
pathogens: Bacterial infections in persons with
human immunodeficiency virus infection. A
review of the literature. *Pharmacotherapy, 13*(6),
543–563.
Glaser, C. A., Angulo, F. J., & Rooney, J. A.
(1994). Animal-associated opportunistic
infections among persons infected with the
human immunodeficiency virus. *Clinical
Infectious Diseases, 18*(1), 14–24.

Syphilis

Katz, D. A., Berger, J. R., & Duncan, R. C. (1993).
Neurosyphilis. A comparative study of the effects
of infection with human immunodeficiency virus.
Archives of Neurology, 50(3), 243–249.
Musher, D. M., Hamill, R. J., & Baughn, R. E.
(1990). Effect of human immunodeficiency virus
(HIV) infection on the course of syphilis and on
the response to treatment. *Annals of Internal
Medicine, 113*(11), 872–881.

Thrombocytopenia

Calenda, V., & Chermann, J. C. (1992). The effects
of HIV on hematopoiesis. *European Journal of
Haematology, 48*(4), 181–186.
Kemeny, M. M., Cooke, V., Melester, T. S.,
Halperin, I. C., Burchell, A. R., Yee, J. P., &
Mills, C. B. (1993). Splenectomy in patients with
AIDS and AIDS-related complex. *AIDS, 7*(8),
1063–1067.
Nydegger, U. E., & Castelli, D. (1991). Review on
therapeutic options in HIV associated
thrombocytopenia with emphasis on i.v.
immunoglobulin treatment. *Immunological
Investigations, 20*(2), 223–229.
Sloand, E. M., Klein, H. G., Banks, S. M.,
Vareldzis, B., Merritt, S., & Pierce, P. (1992).
Epidemiology of thrombocytopenia in HIV
infection. *European Journal of Haematology,
48*(3), 168–172.
Tyler, D. S., Shaunak, S., Bartlett, J. A., & Iglehart,
J. D. (1990). HIV-1–associated
thrombocytopenia. The role of splenectomy.
Annals of Surgery, 211(2), 211–217.

Toxoplasmosis

Bonilla, C. A., & Rosa, U. W. (1994). *Toxoplasma
gondii* pneumonia in patients with the acquired
immunodeficiency syndrome: Diagnosis by
bronchoalveolar lavage. *Southern Medical
Journal, 87*(6), 659–663.
Luft, B. J., & Remington, J. S. (1992). Toxoplasmic
encephalitis in AIDS. *Clinical Infectious
Diseases, 15*(2), 211–222.
Pomeroy, C., & Filice, G. A. (1992). Pulmonary
toxoplasmosis: A review. *Clinical Infectious
Diseases, 14*(4), 863–870.
Stellbrink, H. J., Fuhrer-Burow, R., Raedler, A.,
Albrecht, H., & Fenske, S. (1993). Risk factors
for severe disease due to *Toxoplasma gondii* in
HIV-positive patients. *European Journal of
Epidemiology, 9*(6), 633–637.
Wallace, M. R., Rossetti, R. J., & Olson, P. E. Cats
and toxoplasmosis risk in HIV-infected adults.
JAMA, 269(1), 76–77.

Symptoms and Problems Associated with HIV Disease or Treatment

F

Abdominal Pain

Definition

- Pain resulting from tissue damage to the abdominal viscera or to sympathetically innervated organs

Etiology/Risk Factors

- Ascending cholangitis (CMV infection + cryptosporidiosis)
- Appendicitis
- Cholecystitis
- Enteritis/colitis (usually infectious)
- Organomegaly (tumor, infection)
- Pancreatitis from pentamidine, didanosine (ddI), zalcitabine (ddC), CMV infection
- Perforated viscus (tumor, CMV infection)

Assessment

- Associated symptoms
  - BP changes
  - Diaphoresis
  - Distension
  - Feeling of fullness
  - Heart rate changes
  - Nausea and vomiting
- Cholecystitis and ascending cholangitis: right upper quadrant pain and epigastric pain
- Enteritis/colitis: severe, intense pain; cramping pain associated with diarrhea
- Other types of abdominal pain: vague, deep, dull, aching, squeezing, pressurelike, paroxysmal, colicky
- Pancreatitis: abdominal pain and nausea and vomiting

Diagnostic Tests

- Abdominal CT
- Abdominal radiography
- Serum amylase
- Stool culture

Pharmacologic Management

- Antidiarrheal therapy: kaopectolin, loperamide, diphenoxylate with atropine, paregoric, tincture of opium, octreotride
- Antimicrobial therapy
- Discontinue agents that are producing the pancreatitis
- Opioid analgesics around the clock
- Treatment is directed at the cause of the pain

Nonpharmacologic Management

- Acupuncture
- Distraction
- Hypnosis
- Relaxation and imagery

Potential Problems

- Dehydration
- Depression
- Fatigue
- Nutritional deficit
- Perirectal skin breakdown
- Self-care deficit

Cognitive Impairment

Definition
- Inability to engage in one or more of the following cognitive activities: perception, recognition, conceptualization, judgment, sensation, reason, imagination

Etiology/Risk Factors
- AIDS-dementia complex
- Anxiety
- Aseptic meningitis
- CNS infection
- Cerebrovascular accident
- Depression
- Kaposi's sarcoma
- Lymphoma
- Psychosis
- Side effects of medications

Assessment
- Apathy
- Behavior change
- Change in general appearance
- Decreased attention span
- Difficulty concentrating
- Flat affect
- Forgetfulness
- Inability to perform ADL
- Memory impairments
- Withdrawal behavior
- Withdrawal from social activity

Diagnostic Tests
- CT
- Cultures
- MRI

Pharmacologic Management
- Appropriate antimicrobial therapy
- Neuroleptic agents

Nonpharmacologic Management
- Develop a plan to ensure safety
- Evaluate need for assistive devices (cane, walker)
- Provide cognitive stimulation and orientation
  - Calendar
  - Clock
- Provide written schedule of activities
- Prohibit operation of motor vehicles

Potential Problems
- Depression
- Potential for injury
- Self-care deficit

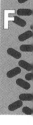

F

Depression: Reactive

Definition
- Depression that occurs in reaction to some outside adverse life situation, usually a crisis or the loss of a person or an established role

Etiology/Risk Factors
- Diagnosis of AIDS
- Fatigue
- Morbidity associated with the disease or treatment
- Pain
- Progression of HIV disease

Assessment
- Anger
- Anorexia
- Constipation
- Discouragement
- Fatigue
- Feelings of guilt
- Feelings of worthlessness
- Insomnia
- Irritability
- Lack of concentration
- Loss of interest and pleasure
- Mild sadness
- Weight loss
- Withdrawal from activities
- Worry

Diagnostic Tests
- None

Pharmacologic Management
- Analgesics (for pain management)
- Selective serotonin reuptake inhibitors
- Tricyclic antidepressants

Nonpharmacologic Management
- Obtain family counseling consultation
- Obtain psychiatric consultation
- Obtain social service referrals
- Structure patient's daily activities

Potential Problems
- Fatigue
- Ineffective family coping
- Self-care deficit
- Suicidal ideation

Diarrhea

Definition
• The passage of frequent stools of a soft or liquid consistency, with or without discomfort

Etiology/Risk Factors
• GI infection
  • Bacteria (e.g., *Salmonella, Shigella, Mycobacterium avium-intracellulare, Campylobacter*)
  • Fungi (e.g., *Candida*)
  • Protozoa (e.g., *Cryptosporidium, Isospora belli, Microsporidium*)
  • Viruses (e.g., CMV, herpes simplex virus)
• GI reaction to medications
• Inappropriate diet therapy
• Intolerance to dietary supplements with high osmolarity
• Kaposi's sarcoma
• Lactose intolerance

Assessment
• Abdominal cramping
• Decreased skin turgor
• Flatus
• Increase in fluid content of stool
• Increase in the number of bowel movements
• Increased bowel sounds

Diagnostic Tests
• BUN
• Intake and output
• Serum creatinine
• Serum electrolytes
• Stool cultures
• Urine specific gravity

Pharmacologic Management

• Antidiarrheal medications on a scheduled basis, not as needed
• Antispasmodic medications

Nonpharmacologic Management

• Avoid anal intercourse and/or oral-anal sexual activities
• Consult with dietician
• Eliminate foods that are irritating or stimulating to the GI tract
• Fecal incontinence pouch for bed-bound patients
• Increase fluid intake to at least 3000 ml/day
• Initiate skin care regimen
• Low-residue, high-protein, high-calorie diet
• Small, frequent meals

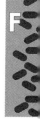

F

Potential Problems
• Dehydration
• Fatigue
• Malnutrition
• Pain
• Perirectal skin breakdown

Dysphagia

Definition
· Difficulty in swallowing

Etiology/Risk Factors
· Alcohol and tobacco use
· Dehydration
· Inadequate oral hygiene
· Malnutrition
· Primary infection of HIV: diffuse infiltrative lymphocytosis syndrome
· Reaction to drug therapy
· Secondary infections
· Bacteria (e.g., *Mycobacterium avium-intracellulare*)
· Fungi (e.g., *Candida albicans*)
· Viruses (e.g., HSV, VZV, varicella zoster)

Assessment
· Choking when swallowing
· Cough reflex
· Coughing while eating
· Cranial nerve functioning
· Food sticking in pharynx or esophagus
· Gag reflex
· Oral cavity assessment
· Pain when swallowing
· Weakness of the oral musculature

Diagnostic Test
· Swallowing assessment

Pharmacologic Management

- Analgesics, parenteral or topical
- Appropriate antibiotic therapy

Nonpharmacologic Management

- Avoid alcohol and tobacco
- Avoid hot, spicy foods
- Begin oral exercises to strengthen lips, jaw, and tongue
- Obtain a consult with a speech pathologist
- Offer frequent, small meals
- Oral hygiene protocol
- Place patient in a sitting or high Fowler's position during and after meals
- Provide dietary supplements

Potential Problems
· Aspiration pneumonia
· Dehydration
· Fatigue
· Nutritional deficit
· Pain

Dyspnea

Definition
• Shortness of breath

Etiology/Risk Factors
• Infection
  • Bacteria (*Mycobacterium tuberculosis,* atypical mycobacteria)
  • Fungi (*Candida albicans, Histoplasma capsulatum, Cryptococcus neoformans*)
  • Protozoa (*Pneumocystis carinii, Cryptosporidium*)
  • Viruses (CMV, HSV)
• Invasion of pulmonary tissue with KS or lymphoma
• Anemia
• Diffuse infiltrative lymphocytosis syndrome
• Exercise intolerance
• Lymphocytic interstitial pneumonitis

Assessment
• Cardiovascular assessment
• Congestion
• Cough
• Fatigue
• Fever
• Pain
• Respiratory assessment
• Sputum production
• Suffocation
• Tightness
• Tingling

Diagnostic Tests
• Arterial blood gases
• Chest radiography
• Pulmonary function tests
• Sputum culture
• Tuberculin skin test

Pharmacologic Management

• Antimicrobial therapy based on culture and sensitivity reports
• Blood transfusion
• Oxygen therapy

Nonpharmacologic Management

• Adequate hydration
• Appropriate body position
• Cognitive therapies to restructure perception of dyspnea
• Coughing and deep-breathing exercises
• Pace activities
• Physical therapy for upper body extremity exercise training
• Pulmonary hygiene measures
• Pursed-lip breathing
• Regular exercise regimen
• Relaxation techniques
• Smoking cessation

Potential Problems
• Anxiety
• Depression
• Immobility
• Infection
• Self-care deficit

F

Fatigue

Definition
- A feeling of weariness, weakness, depletion, and exhaustion or an inability to mobilize energy to carry on that is associated with a desire for sleep and rest

Etiology/Risk factors
- Anemia
- Chronic HIV infection
- Chronic stress
- Diarrhea
- Insomnia
- Malnutrition
- Pain
- Prolonged immobility
- Psychological factors (e.g., depression)
- Secondary opportunistic infection or malignancy

Assessment
- Agitation
- Anorexia
- Apathy
- Decreased ability to make decisions
- Feelings of hopelessness and helplessness
- Impaired concentration and memory
- Insomnia
- Irritability
- Pattern of fatigue
- Tearfulness
- Usual rest and sleep pattern
- Withdrawal

Diagnostic Test
- CBC

Pharmacologic Management
- Transfuse with packed RBCs, if necessary

Nonpharmacologic Management
- Acupressure
- Adequate nutrition
- Adequate sleep
- Develop a rest/activity plan
- Exercise regimen
- Imagery and visualization
- Massage
- Physical therapy consultation
- Progressive muscle relaxation
- Support group participation

Potential Problems
- Depression
- Impaired mobility
- Nutritional deficit
- Suicidal ideation

Fever

Definition
• An elevation of the body temperature above the normal (98.6° F or 37° C)

Etiology/Risk Factors
• Allergic response to medications (drug fever)
• Autoimmune disorders
• Chronic HIV infection
• Dehydration
• Diarrhea
• Infections of IV lines, catheters, drains, incisions
• Malignancy
• Secondary opportunistic infection

Assessment
• Diaphoresis
• Diarrhea
• Disorientation
• Mental status changes
• Rash
• Skin lesions
• Urine color, odor
• Vital signs
• Warm, flushed skin

Diagnostic Tests
• CBC
• Cultures
• Oral temperature
• Urinalysis

Pharmacologic Management

• Analgesics
• Antipyretics
• Appropriate antimicrobial therapy

Nonpharmacologic Management

• Adequate hydration
• Dry clothes and bed linens
• High-protein, high-calorie diet
• Prevent shivering with warm room
• Promote heat loss
• Safety precautions
• Skin care

Potential Problems
• Dehydration
• Fatigue
• Immobility
• Nutritional deficit
• Self-care deficit
• Skin breakdown

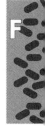

Headache

Definition
- Diffuse pain in various parts of the head

Etiology/Risk Factors
- Aseptic meningitis syndrome
- HSV/HIV encephalitis
- Metastatic KS
- Migraines
- Muscle tension
- Opportunistic viral and nonviral CNS infections
- Primary CNS lymphoma
- Sinus infection
- Toxoplasmosis
- Zidovudine therapy

Assessment
- Cerebral toxoplasmosis: persistent headache that is sometimes associated with focal signs, mental status changes, and seizures
- Encephalitis/meningitis: headache, stiff neck, fever, and other focal neurologic signs
- Neoplasms: headache, focal deficits, weakness, diplopia, blurred vision, personality changes
- Pain assessment
  - Description
  - Location and radiation
  - Severity/intensity
  - Aggravating and relieving factors
  - Previous treatment modalities and effectiveness

Diagnostic Tests
- CBC
- CT
- MRI
- Neurologic examination

Pharmacologic Management

- Low doses of tricyclic antidepressants
- Nonsteroidal antiinflammatory drugs
- Treat the underlying cause of the headache with antimicrobial agents, antineoplastic agents, or radiotherapy

Nonpharmacologic Management

- Biofeedback
- Cold compresses
- Distraction
- Hypnosis
- Relaxation and imagery
- Stress management
- Warm compresses

Potential Problems
- Anxiety
- Depression
- Impaired mobility
- Self-care deficit
- Sleep disturbance

Insomnia

Definition
- Inability to sleep; can be classified into three types: initial (difficulty in falling asleep), intermittent (inability to stay asleep), and terminal (early morning awakening)

Etiology/Risk Factors
- AIDS-dementia complex
- Alcohol dependency
- Anxiety
- Didanosine
- Depression
- Drug dependency
- Stress
- Zidovudine therapy

Assessment
- Alcohol and drug history
- Anxiety
- Depression
- Irritability
- Loss of train of thought
- Mental confusion
- Number and timing of naps
- Usual sleep pattern
  - Intrusive thoughts
  - Number of awakenings
  - Time of morning awakening
  - Time needed to fall asleep
  - Time of retirement
  - Total sleep time

Diagnostic Tests
- None

Pharmacologic Management

- Use appropriate medications to provide symptomatic relief and enhance sleep
  - Antianxiety medications
  - Antihistamines
  - Hypnotics
  - Psychotropic drugs
  - Sedatives
  - Tricyclic antidepressants
- Benzodiazepines may alter the pharmacokinetics of zidovudine and increase toxicity

Nonpharmacologic Management

- Avoid excessive stimulation at bedtime
- Drink a warm liquid containing milk before bedtime
- Engage in restful activities before bedtime
- Establish regular time for sleep
- Establish regular sleep routine
- Relaxation exercises

F

Potential Problems
- Cognitive impairment
- Confusion
- Depression
- Fatigue

Myalgia

Definition
- Muscle pain

Etiology/Risk Factors
- Acute HIV infection
- Dermatomyositis
- Polymyositis
- Zidovudine therapy

Assessment
- Atrophy
- Fasciculations
- Muscle pain
  - Description
  - Location
  - Severity/intensity
  - Aggravating and relieving factors
  - Previous treatment modalities and effectiveness
- Weakness

Diagnostic Test
- EMG

Pharmacologic Management

- Nonopioid analgesics
- Nonsteroidal antiinflammatory drugs

Nonpharmacologic Management

- Application of warm or cold compresses
- Exercise regimen
- Hypnosis
- Massage
- Relaxation and imagery

Potential Problems
- Fatigue
- Impaired mobility
- Self-care deficit

Peripheral Neuropathy

Definition

· Constant or intermittent burning, aching, or lancinating limb pain due to generalized or focal diseases of peripheral nerves

Etiology/Risk Factors

· CMV radiculitis
· Didanosine (ddI)
· Herpes zoster radiculitis
· Infiltration of nerves with lymphoma
· Postherpetic neuralgia
· Vitamin B deficiency
· Vitamin E deficiency
· Zalcitabine (ddC)

Assessment

· Allodynia
· Atrophy
· Diminished reflexes
· Distal weakness
· Hyperalgesia
· Pain
  · Aching
  · Burning
  · Disesthesias
  · Sharp, lancinating
· Stocking-glove sensory loss

Diagnostic Tests

· EMG
· Somatosensory testing

Pharmacologic Management

· Anticonvulsants (for stabbing, shocklike pain)
  · Carbamazepine 200–1600 mg/day PO
  · Phenytoin 300–500 mg/day PO
· Antidepressants
  · Amitriptyline 25–150 mg/day PO
  · Doxepin 25–150 mg/day PO
  · Imipramine 20–100 mg/day PO
  · Trazadone 75–225 mg/day PO
· Local anesthesia
  · Mexiletine 450–600 mg/day PO
  · Tocainide 20 mg/kg/day PO
· Retroviral therapy (zidovudine)
· Treat the underlying infections or neoplasms

Nonpharmacologic Management

· Acupuncture
· Distraction
· Hypnosis
· Relaxation and imagery
· TENS

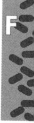

Potential Problems

· Depression
· Fatigue
· Impaired mobility
· Potential for injury
· Self-care deficit

Visual Disturbances

Definition
• Changes in visual acuity as a result of a disease process

Etiology/Risk Factors
• AIDS-related microangiopathy
• HIV infection of the eye
• KS
• Lymphoma
• Ocular infection
  • Bacteria (e.g., *Mycobacterium avium-intracellulare*)
  • Fungi (e.g., *Cryptococcus neoformans, Histoplasma capsulatum, Candida albicans*)
  • Protozoa (e.g., *Toxoplasma gondii, Pneumocystis carinii*)
  • Viruses (e.g., CMV, HSV, herpes zoster)
• Side effects of medications

Assessment
• Emotional impact of visual disturbances
• Examination of cranial nerve function
  • Abducens (VI)
  • Oculomotor (III)
  • Optic (II)
  • Trigeminal (V)
  • Trochlear (IV)
• Limitations on ADL imposed by visual disturbances
• Visual acuity
  • Blurred vision
  • Floaters
  • Gaps in vision
• Visual impairments

Diagnostic Tests
• Ophthalmoscopic examination
• Snellen chart

Pharmacologic Management
• Appropriate antimicrobial therapy

Nonpharmacologic Management
• Develop plan to ensure safety in the home
• Minimize sensitivity to bright lights
• Occupational therapy consult
• Ophthamology consult
• Referral to local organization for the blind

Potential Problems
• Anxiety
• Depression
• Potential for injury
• Self-care deficit

Weight Loss

Definition
· Decrease in body weight below ideal body weight

Etiology/Risk Factors
· Alterations in taste
· Anorexia
· Catabolic processes
· Depression
· Diarrhea
· Dysphagia
· Fatigue
· Fever
· Hypermetabolism
· Impaired chewing
· Impaired cognition
· Malabsorption
· Nausea and vomiting
· Pain

Assessment
· Current medication profile
· Current weight
· Dietary history
· Economic resources to buy, store, and prepare food
· Mental status and cognitive status

Diagnostic Tests
· Anthropometric measurements
· CBC
· Iron-binding capacity
· Serum albumin
· Serum cholesterol
· Serum triglycerides
· Swallowing assessment
· Total protein

Pharmacologic Management

· High-protein, high-calorie diet
· Nutritional supplements (e.g., Isocal, Ensure, Ensure Plus, Carnation Instant Breakfast)

Nonpharmacologic Management

· Appropriate referrals (e.g., Meals on Wheels)
· Consult with dietician
· Dental consult
· Eliminate nonnutritious food
· Exercise program
· Oral care regimen
· Small, frequent meals

Potential Problems
· Decreased mobility
· Depression
· Fatigue
· Infections
· Self-care deficit

F

Bibliography

Abdominal Pain

Bonacini, M., & Skodras, G. (1993). Gastrointestinal endoscopic pathology in patients seropositive for human immunodeficiency virus. *Missouri Medicine, 90*(2), 85–89.

Mueller, G. P., & Williams, R. A. (1995). Surgical infections in AIDS patients. *American Journal of Surgery, 169*(5A, Suppl.), 34S–38S.

Rosengart, T. K., & Coppa, G. F. (1990). Abdominal mycobacterial infections in immunocompromised patients. *American Journal of Surgery, 59*(1), 125–131.

Depression

Judd, F. K., & Mijch, A. M. (1994). Depression in patients with HIV and AIDS. *Australian and New Zealand Journal of Psychiatry, 28*(4), 642–650.

Diarrhea

Bonacini, M., & Skodras, G. (1993). Gastrointestinal endoscopic pathology in patients seropositive for human immunodeficiency virus. *Missouri Medicine, 90*(2), 85–89.

Dieterich, D. T., & Rahmin M. (1991). Cytomegalovirus colitis in AIDS: Presentation in 44 patients and a review of the literature. *Journal of Acquired Immune Deficiency Syndromes, 4*(Suppl. 1), S29–S35.

Simon, D., Weiss, L. M., & Brandt, L. J. (1992). Treatment options for AIDS-related esophageal and diarrheal disorders. *American Journal of Gastroenterology, 87*(3), 274–281.

Dysphagia

Laguna, F., Garcia-Samaniego, J., Soriano, V., Valencia, E., Redondo, C., Alonso, M. J., & Gonzalez-Lahoz, J. M. (1994). Gastrointestinal leishmaniasis in human immunodeficiency virus–infected patients: Report of five cases and review. *Clinical Infectious Diseases, 19*(1), 48–53.

Dyspnea

Hurley, P. M., & Ungvarski, P. J. (1994). Home healthcare needs of adults living with HIV disease/AIDS in New York City. *Journal of the Association of Nurses in Aids Care, 5*(2), 33–40.

Fatigue

Levinson, S. F., & O'Connell, P. G. (1991). Rehabilitation dimensions of AIDS: A review. *Archives of Physical Medicine and Rehabilitation, 72*(9), 690–696.

Whalen, C. C., Antani, M., Carey, J., & Landefeld, C. S. (1994). An index of symptoms for infection with human immunodeficiency virus: Reliability and validity. *Journal of Clinical Epidemiology, 47*(5), 537–546.

Fever

Hambleton, J., Aragon, T., Modin, G., Northfelt, D. W., & Sande, M. A. (1995). Outcome for hospitalized patients with fever and neutropenia who are infected with the human immunodeficiency virus. *Clinical Infectious Diseases, 20*(2), 363–371.

Weisse, A. B., Heller, D. R., Schimenti, R. J., Montgomery, R. L., & Kapila, R. (1993). The febrile parenteral drug user: A prospective study in 121 patients. *American Journal of Medicine, 94*(3), 274–80.

Headache

Holloway, R. G., & Kieburtz, K. D. (1995). Headache and the human immunodeficiency virus type 1 infection. *Headache, 35*(5), 245–255.

Insomnia

Ochitill, H., Dilley, J., & Kohlwes, J. (1991). Psychotropic drug prescribing for hospitalized patients with acquired immunodeficiency syndrome. *American Journal of Medicine, 90*(5), 601–605.

Peripheral Neuropathy

Brew, B. J. (1994). The clinical spectrum and pathogenesis of HIV encephalopathy, myelopathy, and peripheral neuropathy. *Current Opinion in Neurology, 7*(3), 209–216.

Tyor, W. R., Wesselingh, S. L., Griffin, J. W., McArthur, J. C., & Griffin, D. E. (1995). Unifying hypothesis for the pathogenesis of HIV-associated dementia complex, vacuolar myelopathy, and sensory neuropathy. *Journal of Acquired Immune Deficiency Syndromes and Human Retrovirology, 9*(4), 379–388.

Visual Disturbances

Agbeja, A. M., & Cookey-Gam, A. I. (1992). Rehabilitation of the blind: A review. *East African Medical Journal, 69*(6), 341–344.

Ugen, K. E., McCallus, D. E., Von Feldt, J. M., Williams, W. V., Greene, M. I., & Weiner, D. B. (1992). Ocular tissue involvement in HIV infection: Immunological and pathological aspects. *Immunologic Research, 11*(2), 141–153.

Weight Loss

Coodley, G. O., Loveless, M. O., & Merrill, T. M. (1994). The HIV wasting syndrome: A review. *Journal of Acquired Immune Deficiency Syndromes, 7*(7), 681–694.

Keusch, G. T., & Thea, D. M. (1993). Malnutrition in AIDS. *Medical Clinics of North America, 77*(4), 795–814.

McKinley, M. J., Goodman-Block, J., Lesser, M. L., & Salbe, A. D. (1994). Improved body weight status as a result of nutrition intervention in adult, HIV-positive outpatients. *Journal of the American Dietetic Association, 94*(9), 1014–1017.

Nahlen, B. L., Chu, S. Y., Nwanyanwu, O. C., Berkelman, R. L., Martinez, S. A., & Rullan, J. V. (1993). HIV wasting syndrome in the United States. *AIDS, 7*(2), 183–188.

Zangerle, R., Reibnegger, G., Wachter, H., & Fuchs, D. (1993). Weight loss in HIV-1 infection is associated with immune activation. *AIDS, 7*(2), 175–181.

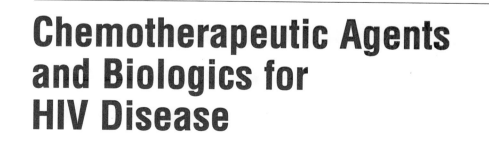

Chemotherapeutic Agents and Biologics for HIV Disease

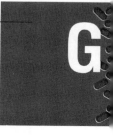

G

Acyclovir (Zovirax)

Drug Classification
Antiviral agent

Mechanism
• Interferes with viral DNA synthesis

Administration
• PO, IV, topical

Therapeutic Use
• Epstein-Barr virus
• Hairy leukoplakia
• HSV
• VZV

Usual Dose and Schedule

• Initial genital herpes: 200 mg PO q4h while awake for 10 days, or 5 mg/kg IV q8h for 5 days
• Chronic therapy for recurrent genital herpes: 400 mg PO b.i.d. for up to 12 months
• Acute treatment of herpes zoster: 800 mg PO q4h while awake for 7–10 days
• Chickenpox: 20 mg/kg PO q.i.d. for 5 days (not to exceed 800 mg/dose)
• Mucosal and cutaneous herpes simplex in immunocompromised patients: 5 mg/kg IV q8h for 7 days
• Herpes simplex encephalitis: 10 mg/kg IV q8h for 10 days

Side Effects/Toxicities
• Arthralgias
• Diarrhea
• Dizziness
• Headache
• Joint pain
• Nausea and vomiting
• Pain at injection site
• Phlebitis
• Renal failure

Special Considerations
• Capsules should be taken with meals
• If taken in combination with zidovudine severe drowsiness and lethargy may occur
• Take medication for the full course of therapy

Atovaquone (Acuvel, BW-566C80, Mepron)

Drug Classification
Antiprotozoal

Administration
• PO

Therapeutic Use
• *Pneumocystis carinii* pneumonia

Mechanism
• Inhibits the action of enzymes necessary to nucleic acid and adenosine triphosphate synthesis in protozoa

Usual Dose and Schedule

• 750 mg PO t.i.d. for 21 days

Side Effects/Toxicities
• Diarrhea
• Fever
• Headache
• Hepatotoxicity
• Insomnia
• Nausea and vomiting
• Rash
• Weakness

Special Considerations
• Second-line therapy for PCP
• Administer with food to increase absorption

G

Azithromycin (Zithromax)

Drug Classification
Macrolide antibiotic

Mechanism
• Inhibits protein synthesis

Administration
• PO

Therapeutic Use
• *Mycobacterium avium-intracellulare*
• Nongonococcal urethritis and cervicitis

Usual Dose and Schedule

• 500 mg on day 1, then 250 mg/day for 4 more days (total dose 1.5 g)

Side Effects/Toxicities
• Abdominal pain
• Diarrhea
• Dizziness
• Headache
• Nausea
• Ototoxicity

Special Considerations
• Aluminum or magnesium antacids may alter absorption
• Take on an empty stomach

Clarithromycin (Biaxin)

Drug Classification
Macrolide antibiotic

Mechanism
· Inhibits protein synthesis

Administration
· PO

Therapeutic Use
· *Mycobacterium avium-intracellulare*

Usual Dose and Schedule
· 500–1000 mg q12h

Side Effects/Toxicities
· Abnormal taste sensation
· Diarrhea
· Headache
· Nausea
· Ototoxicity

Special Considerations
· Adjust dose for renal disease

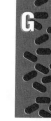

G

Dapsone (DDS)

Drug Classification
Antimicrobial, leprostatic agent

Mechanism
• Exact mechanism of action is unknown

Administration
• PO

Therapeutic Use
• Leprosy
• Second-line treatment or prophylaxis for PCP

Usual Dose

- PCP treatment: 100 mg/day PO for 21 days
- PCP prophylaxis: 50–100 mg/day PO once a day to 3 times per week

Side Effects/Toxicities
• Abdominal pain
• Abnormal liver function tests
• Agranulocytosis
• Blurred vision
• Headache
• Hemolytic anemia
• Insomnia
• Methemoglobinemia
• Nausea/vomiting
• Peripheral neuropathy
• Phototoxicity
• Rash
• Vertigo

Special Considerations
• Rifampin decreases serum levels of dapsone
• Didanosine decreases dapsone absorption

Didanosine (DDI, dideoxyinosine, Videx)

Drug Classification
Antimicrobial, antiretroviral agent

Mechanism
· Inhibits viral replication by interfering with viral RNA–directed DNA polymerase

Administration
· PO, buffered powder for an oral solution

Therapeutic Use
· HIV infection

Usual Dose and Schedule

· Adults ($\geq$ 60 kg) 200 mg PO b.i.d.
· Adults ($<$ 60 kg) 125 mg PO b.i.d.

Side Effects/Toxicities
· Anemia
· Chills
· Cough
· Diarrhea
· Fever
· Headache
· Hepatitis
· Hyperuricemia
· Insomnia
· Leukopenia
· Myalgia
· Nausea and vomiting
· Pancreatitis
· Peripheral neuropathy
· Rhinitis
· Seizures

Special Considerations
· Decreases absorption of dapsone; the two drugs must be taken two hours apart
· Decrease dose in patients with renal dysfunction

G

Foscarnet (Foscavir)

Drug Classification
Antimicrobial, antiretroviral, antiviral

Mechanism
- Prevents viral replication by inhibiting viral DNA polymerase and reverse transcriptase

Administration
- IV

Therapeutic Use
- Acyclovir-resistant herpes
- CMV

Usual Dose and Schedule

- Induction: 60 mg/kg IV q8h for 14–21 days
- Maintenance: 90–120 mg/kg/day IV

Side Effects/Toxicities
- Acute renal failure
- Anemia
- Arthralgia
- Diarrhea
- Fever
- Genital ulcers
- Headache
- Hyper-/hypocalcemia
- Hyper-/hypophosphatemia
- Hypokalemia
- Hypomagnesemia
- Myalgia
- Nausea
- Neutropenia
- Paresthesias
- Renal failure
- Seizures
- Thrombocytopenia

Special Considerations
- Reduce dose in patients with impaired renal function
- Inform patient that foscarnet is not a cure for CMV retinitis

Ganciclovir (Cytovene)

Drug Classification
Antimicrobial, antiviral

Mechanism
• Inhibits viral DNA polymerase

Administration
• IV, intravitreal

Therapeutic Use
• Acyclovir-resistant herpes
• CMV infection
• CMV prophylaxis in patients receiving an organ transplant
• CMV retinitis

Usual Dose and Schedule

• Induction: 5.0 mg/kg IV q12h for 14–21 days
• Maintenance: 5.0 mg/kg IV 7 days/week or 6.0 mg/kg IV 5 days/week
• Intravitreal: 200 µg once weekly

Side Effects/Toxicities
• Confusion
• Headache
• Increased liver enzymes
• Neutropenia
• Phlebitis
• Rash
• Retinal detachment
• Seizures
• Thrombocytopenia

Special Considerations
• Adjust dose in patients with renal disease
• Monitor absolute neutrophil count and platelet count
• Consider placement of a central line
• Ophthamology consult

G

Interferon Alfa-2a

Drug Classification
Immunoregulating agent

Mechanism
• Antiviral activity

Administration
• IM, SC

Therapeutic Use
• AIDS-related KS

Usual Dose and Schedule

• 36 million IU/day for 10–12 weeks or 3 million IU/day for 3 days, then 9 million IU/day for next 3 days, then 18 million IU/day for next 3 days, then 36 million IU/day for rest of 10–12 week course
• Maintenance dose of 36 million IU, 3 times a week

Side Effects/Toxicities
• Alopecia
• Altered taste
• Anemia
• Anorexia
• Chills
• Depression
• Diarrhea
• Dry mouth
• Edema
• Fatigue
• Fever
• Flulike syndrome
• Hypotension
• Impotence
• Leukopenia
• Myalgia
• Nausea
• Pruritus
• Rash
• Sleep disturbance
• Thrombocytopenia
• Vomiting
• Weight loss

Special Considerations
• Monitor number, size, and character of KS lesions before and during therapy
• SC route preferred for patients with a platelet count $< 50,000/\mu m$

Ribavirin (Virazole)

Drug Classification
Antiviral

Mechanism
- Inhibits viral DNA and RNA synthesis and replication

Administration
- Inhalation

Therapeutic Use
- Treatment of severe lower respiratory tract infection caused by the respiratory syncytial virus in infants and children

Usual Dose and Schedule
- 300 ml of 200-mg/ml solution delivered through mist for 12–18 hours/day

Side Effects/Toxicities
- Blurred vision
- Cardiac arrest
- Dizziness
- Faintness
- Hypotension
- Ocular irritation
- Photosensitivity
- Rash
- Reticulocytosis

Special Considerations
- May antagonize action of zidovudine

G

Stavudine (D4T, Zerit)

Drug Classification
Antiretroviral

Mechanism
- Nucleoside analog that inhibits viral replication

Administration
- PO

Therapeutic Use
- Failure of or intolerance to other antiretroviral drugs

Usual Dose and Schedule

- Adults (< 60 kg) 30 mg PO b.i.d.
- Adults (> 60 kg) 40 mg PO b.i.d.

Side Effects/Toxicities
- Granulocytopenia
- Headache
- Hepatotoxicity
- Hyperamylanemia
- Myelosuppression
- Myopathy
- Pancreatitis
- Peripheral neuropathy

Special Considerations
- Adjust dose in patients with renal impairment or if peripheral neuropathy develops
- Do not combine with zidovudine

Zalcitabine (ddC, dideoxycytidine, Hivid)

Drug Classification
Antimicrobial, antiretroviral

Mechanism
- Inhibits viral DNA synthesis and replication
- Nucleoside analog that inhibits the enzyme reverse transcriptase

Administration
- PO

Therapeutic Use
- HIV infection

Usual Dose and Schedule
- 0.375 mg or 0.75 mg PO t.i.d.

Side Effects/Toxicities
- Cardiomyopathy
- Congestive heart failure
- Fever
- Headache
- Malaise
- Oral ulcers
- Pancreatitis
- Peripheral neuropathy
- Rash
- Weight loss

Special Considerations
- Decrease dose in patients with impaired renal function
- Discontinue therapy in patients who develop peripheral neuropathy, and restart at 50% of previous dose

G

Zidovudine (azidothymidine, AZT, Retrovir, ZDV)

Drug Classification
Antiretroviral

Mechanism
- Inhibits viral RNA synthesis by inhibiting the enzyme DNA polymerase
- Prevents viral replication

Administration
- PO, IV

Therapeutic Use
- HIV infection

Usual Dose and Schedule

- Symptomatic HIV infection: 100 mg PO q4h; 1–2 mg/kg infused over 1 hour q4h
- Asymptomatic HIV infection: 100 mg PO q4h while awake (500 mg/day)

Side Effects/Toxicities
- Abdominal pain
- Anemia
- Diarrhea
- Fatigue
- Granulocytopenia
- Headache
- Myopathy
- Nausea and vomiting
- Weakness

Special Considerations
- Administer medication around the clock
- Monitor for anemia (usually occurs within 2–4 weeks) and granulocytopenia (usually occurs within 6–8 weeks)
- Must be taken with food

Bibliography

Acyclovir

Adair, J. C., Gold, M., & Bond, R. E. (1994). Acyclovir neurotoxicity: Clinical experience and review of the literature. *Southern Medical Journal, 87*(12), 1227–1231.

Coen, D. M. (1994). Acyclovir-resistant, pathogenic herpes viruses. *Trends in Microbiology, 2*(12), 481–485.

Rothe, M. J., Feder, H. M., Jr., & Grant-Kels, J. M. (1991). Oral acyclovir therapy for varicella and zoster infections in pediatric and pregnant patients: A brief review. *Pediatric Dermatology, 8*(3), 236–242, 246–247.

Wood, M. J. (1994). Current experience with antiviral therapy for acute herpes zoster. *Annals of Neurology, 35*(Suppl.), S65–S68.

Atovaquone

Haile, L. G., & Flaherty, J. F. (1993). Atovaquone: A review. *Annals of Pharmacotherapy, 27*(12), 1488–1494.

Azithromycin

Bahal, N., & Nahata, M. C. (1992). The new macrolide antibiotics: Azithromycin, clarithromycin, dirithromycin, and roxithromycin. *Annals of Pharmacology, 26*(1), 46–55.

Goldman, M. P., & Longworth, D. L. (1993). The role of azithromycin and clarithromycin in clinical practice. *Cleveland Clinic Journal of Medicine, 60*(5), 359–364.

Kissinger, P., Clark, R., Morse, A., & Brandon, W. (1995). Comparison of multiple drug therapy regimens for HIV-related disseminated *Mycobacterium avium* complex disease. *Journal of Acquired Immune Deficiency Syndromes and Human Retrovirology, 9*(2), 133–137.

Periti, P., Mazzei, T., Mini, E., & Novelli, A. (1993). Adverse effects of macrolide antibacterials. *Drug Safety, 9*(5), 346–364.

Peters, D. H., Friedel, H. A., & McTavish, D. (1992). Azithromycin. A review of its antimicrobial activity, pharmacokinetic properties and clinical efficacy. *Drugs, 44*(5), 750–799.

Rapp, R. P., McCraney, S. A., Goodman, N. L., & Shaddick, D. J. (1994). New macrolide antibiotics: Usefulness in infections caused by mycobacteria other than mycobacterium tuberculosis. *Annals of Pharmacotherapy, 28*(11), 1255–1263.

Clarithromycin

Barradell, L. B., Plosker, G. L., & McTavish, D. (1993). Clarithromycin. A review of its pharmacological properties and therapeutic use in *Mycobacterium avium-intracellulare* complex infection in patients with acquired immune deficiency syndrome. *Drugs, 46*(2), 289–312.

Dempsey, C. L., Kaley, T. C., & Zenkel, J. (1993). Drug usage evaluation: Clarithromycin as sequential therapy. *Hospital Formulary, 28*(12), 999–1001.

Hardy, D. J., Guay, D. R., & Jones, R. N. (1992). Clarithromycin, a unique macrolide. A pharmacokinetic, microbiological, and clinical overview. *Diagnostic Microbiology and Infectious Disease, 15*(1), 39–53.

Peters, D. H., & Clissold, S. P. (1992). Clarithromycin. A review of its antimicrobial activity, pharmacokinetic properties and therapeutic potential. *Drugs, 44*(1), 117–164.

Sturgill, M. G., & Rapp, R. P. (1992). Clarithromycin: Review of a new macrolide antibiotic with improved microbiologic spectrum and favorable pharmacokinetic and adverse effect profiles. *Annals of Pharmacotherapy, 26*(9), 1099–1108.

Dapsone

Hansen, D. G., Challoner, K. R., & Smith, D. E. (1994). Dapsone intoxication: Two case reports. *Journal of Emergency Medicine, 12*(3), 347–351.

Kemper, C. A., Tucker, R. M., Lang, O. S., Kessinger, J. M., Greene, S. I., Deresinski, S. C., & Stevens, D. A. (1990). Low-dose dapsone prophylaxis of *Pneumocystis carinii* pneumonia in AIDS and AIDS-related complex. *AIDS, 4*(11), 1145–1148.

Pertel, P., & Hirschtick, R. (1994). Adverse reactions to dapsone in persons infected with human immunodeficiency virus. *Clinical Infectious Diseases, 18*(4), 630–632.

Didanosine

Faulds, D., & Brogden, R. N. (1992). Didanosine. A review of its antiviral activity, pharmacokinetic properties and therapeutic potential in human immunodeficiency virus infection. *Drugs, 44*(1), 94–116.

Franssen, R. M., Meenhorst, P. L., Koks, C. H., & Beijnen, J. H. (1992). Didanosine, a new antiretroviral drug. A review. *Pharmaceutisch Weekblad. Scientific Edition, 4*(5), 297–304.

Liebman, H. A., & Cooley, T. P. (1993). Didanosine in the treatment of AIDS and AIDS-related complex: A critical appraisal of the dose and frequency of administration. *Clinical Infectious Diseases, 16*(Suppl. 1), S52–S58.

Morse, G. D., Shelton, M. J., & O'Donnell, A. M. (1993). Comparative pharmacokinetics of antiviral nucleoside analogues. *Clinical Pharmacokinetics, 24*(2), 101–123.

Rathbun, R. C., & Martin, E. S., 3d. (1992). Didanosine therapy in patients intolerant of or failing zidovudine therapy. *Annals of Pharmacotherapy, 26*(11), 1347–1351.

Shelton, M. J., O'Donnell, A. M., & Morse, G. D. (1992). Didanosine. *Annals of Pharmacotherapy, 26*(5), 660–670.

Foscarnet

Chrisp, P., & Clissold, S. P. (1991). Foscarnet. A review of its antiviral activity, pharmacokinetic properties and therapeutic use in immunocompromised patients with cytomegalovirus retinitis. *Drugs, 41*(1), 104–129.

Fanning, M. M., Read, S. E., Benson, M., Vas, S., Rachlis, A., Kozousek, V., Mortimer, C., Harvey, P., Schwartz, C., & Chew, E. (1990). Foscarnet therapy of cytomegalovirus retinitis in AIDS. *Journal of Acquired Immune Deficiency Syndromes, 3*(5), 472–479.

Jacobson, M. A. (1992). Review of the toxicities of foscarnet. *Journal of Acquired Immune Deficiency Syndromes, 5*(Suppl. 1), S11–S17.

Ganciclovir

Faulds, D., & Heel, R. C. (1990). Ganciclovir. A review of its antiviral activity, pharmacokinetic properties and therapeutic efficacy in cytomegalovirus infections. *Drugs, 39*(4), 597–638.

Morley, M. G., Duker, J. S., Ashton, P., & Robinson, M. R. (1995). Replacing ganciclovir implants. *Ophthalmology, 102*(3), 388–392.

Interferon

Dorr, R. T. (1993). Interferon-alpha in malignant and viral diseases. A review. *Drugs, 45*(2), 177–211.

Pitha, P. M. (1994). Multiple effects of interferon on the replication of human immunodeficiency virus type 1. *Antiviral Research, 24*(2–3), 205–219.

Stein, D. S., Timpone, J. G., Gradon, J. D., Kagan, J. M., & Schnittman, S. M. (1993). Immune-based therapeutics: Scientific rationale and the promising approaches to the treatment of the human immunodeficiency virus–infected

G

individual. *Clinical Infectious Diseases, 17*(4), 749–771.

Ribavirin

Feldstein, T. J., Swegarden, J. L., Atwood, G. F., & Peterson, C. D. (1995). Ribavirin therapy: Implementation of hospital guidelines and effect on usage and cost of therapy. *Pediatrics, 96*(1, Pt. 1), 14–17.

Knight, V., Gilbert, B. E., Wyde, P. R., & Englund, J. A. (1991). High dose–short duration ribavirin aerosol treatment—a review. *Bulletin of the International Union Against Tuberculosis and Lung Disease, 66*(2–3), 97–101.

Zalcitabine

Shelton, M. J., O'Donnell, A. M., & Morse, G. D. (1993). Zalcitabine. *Annals of Pharmacotherapy, 27*(4), 480–489.

Whittington, R., & Brogden, R. N. (1992). Zalcitabine. A review of its pharmacology and clinical potential in acquired immunodeficiency syndrome (AIDS). *Drugs, 4*(4), 656–683.

Zidovudine

Brouker, M. E., Donegan, S. E., Karney, W. W., & Mayers, D. L. (1990). An updated therapeutic review. Zidovudine. *Navy Medicine, 81*(1), 26–28.

Hoover, D. R. (1995). The effects of long term zidovudine therapy and *pneumocystis carinii* prophylaxis on HIV disease. A review of the literature. *Drugs, 49*(1), 20–36.

Rachlis, A. R. (1990). Zidovudine (Retrovir) update. *Canadian Medical Association Journal, 143*(11), 1177–1185.

Index

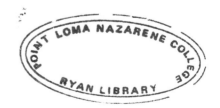